CW00733670

Adventures In Anaesthesia

By

Dr Ellie May

Adventures in Anaesthesia

Copyright © Dr Ellie May
September 2014

This book is based on my experiences in hospital medicine as I began training in anaesthesia. Names, events, locations and gender have each been changed to ensure the anonymity of doctors and confidentiality of patients involved are maintained. The facts remain true. The descriptions of my hospital workplaces are accurate but my recollection of events and opinions of healthcare systems and services are my own.

1. The End of the Beginning

'Anaesthetic registrar to resus. Anaesthetic registrar to resus.'

The call crackled from my bleep waking me from my deep slumber at 2am. Typically, it was my last night on call.

I jumped out of bed, already dressed in theatre clothes doubling as pyjamas. I rushed to the resuscitation room in accident and emergency as instructed, not stopping to brush my teeth or hair.

Kirsty was sat bolt upright gasping for air. The high flow oxygen was whistling as it sped through the chamber filled with adrenaline, carrying it into her mouth.

'Hi' said the casualty doctor. 'Peanut allergy.' he nodded to indicate our patient. 'Been in about an hour. Getting worse rather than better I'm afraid'

I introduced myself to Kirsty. She had clearly come straight from a party: her red dress looked expensive, despite the patches of sweat developing. The colour was strong and vibrant in the stark contrast to her profound pallor. Her matching shoes, heels of crazy proportions, had been discarded and now lay redundant under the trolley.

She was braced against the rails of the trolley, arms rigid. Her hair was plastered to her face, her neck muscles taut, the veins bulging as she concentrated on drawing the next breath. She acknowledged me with a nod, not wasting any precious breath on unnecessary small talk. I learned she had been at a friend's 21st birthday party. She enjoyed the buffet, choosing carefully as she always did, to avoid anything which may contain peanuts. It was too late when she realised the skewered chicken was in fact chicken satay. Her tongue was immediately tingly and recognising the sign, she self-administered her ever present Epipen, delivering adrenaline swiftly into her thigh to halt the reaction.

Despite her swift action she was now paying the price. Her tongue was progressively swelling such that her speech was slurred and indistinct, as if inebriated.

The swelling was not confined to the tongue. It was spreading to the palate above and towards the back of her throat. Her airway, that lifeline from the nose and mouth down to the lungs, was narrowing rapidly. The other signs of anaphylaxis were all there too. The facial flush, the low blood pressure and the rising heart rate. Her pupils were wild and dilated, a combination of fear and adrenaline. Adrenaline both nebulised from the chamber and from her own body's fight or flight response being maximally activated.

She needed urgent intubation to place a breathing tube into her windpipe to protect her airway from complete occlusion. Passing a tube through the mouth, down the back of the throat, through the vocal cords and into the trachea, would ensure the safe transit of oxygen and air to the lungs, but would be no mean feat. A swollen airway can rapidly be fatal and fills most anaesthetists with fear. I was no different.

I transferred her to the operating theatre where I had skilled help and specialised equipment. I called my consultant. The grumpy old sod needed to retire and would be none too pleased being awoken at this time of night. Despite this and knowing he was 30 minutes away, I asked him to attend. He was still the boss after all and I was long past being intimidated by his bad temper. Next I called the Ear, Nose and Throat consultant and was relieved that he was closer and much more pleasant. He was my get out of jail free card.

After quickly preparing the drugs I would require and checking the equipment, I explained to Kirsty that I needed to put her off to sleep and protect her airway with a breathing tube to keep her alive while the swelling ran its course, threatening to engulf and overwhelm her upper airway.

'If I am unable to safely maneuver the tube into the correct position, my ENT colleague is here to cut emergency access into your windpipe via the front of your neck' It sounded barbaric and I didn't mince my words. It is a serious business. Emergency tracheostomy is a life saving surgical procedure to provide a patent airway for patients in the last chance saloon.

She nodded in consent to the proposed procedures. What option did she have?

I started with plan A. Holding the clear plastic mask firmly onto her face, covering both her nose and mouth I spoke quietly in an effort to calm her and instructed her to take slow deep breaths. Gradually, I added some anaesthetic gas into the oxygen she breathed. This meant anaesthesia was induced very slowly, her breaths reduced by the partially obstructed airway, but it preserved her own spontaneous breathing effort, sustaining life for as long as possible.

Ten minutes later I decided she was anaesthetised deeply enough to look into her mouth. My hands were shaking, my knuckles white through a combination of fear and gripping the face mask tightly to her face, lending support to her airway as the accessory breathing muscles in her neck relaxed and she lost consciousness.

With a nod to the anaesthetic nurse assisting me, I was handed the shiny cold stainless steel laryngoscope. I inserted it as usual, down the right hand side of the tongue. I advanced it towards the back of her throat while listening for the sound and feel of it clunking into the vallecula, that valley between the back of the tongue and the epiglottis. The clunk never came. The monitor continued to bleep, the only sound in theatre at that moment.

The tissues inside her mouth were red and amorphous, swollen such that normal anatomy was distorted. I lifted the laryngoscope with the superman arm action required, desperate to see the familiar leaf shaped epiglottis standing proud above the white vocal cords, protecting them and signalling the entrance to the airway. I wanted to see where I needed to place the tube.

Nothing was recognisable. I could not see the epiglottis nor anything else I recognised for that matter. The airway was a spongy mass engulfing the blade of the laryngoscope, bulging at every point, obscuring my view.

The tongue was engorged and too voluminous to displace to the left of the mouth and allow a view beyond the tonsils.

'If in doubt, come out'. An anaesthetic mantra sprang to mind.

I removed the blade from her mouth and returned the mask to her face, with the oxygen flow dialled up to maximum. With relief I saw the reservoir bag filling and emptying, a visible sign her spontaneous breathing remained and my intervention had not precipitated reactionary closure of the airways.

I considered my findings and debated my plan B. Trying again was likely to be futile and may precipitate a disastrous deterioration. Using a fibre-optic scope to navigate through the swollen airway would be difficult and I would need more than just my own two hands to do this whilst simultaneously propping the airway open to allow breathing to continue.

Just then, my consultant walked into theatre. The relief this brought was almost palpable. I could hear the sigh, a collective exhalation from all the theatre staff as they relaxed, their tension eased now the consultant was present. I aspired to have this effect on a situation.

'What's the case here?' he rubbed his hands together as if in delight. He seemed in a surprisingly good mood. I decided it was a good omen. 'Don't mind me, looks like you're doing an excellent job'.

I was not convinced of this, but filled him in on the history and my initial recent examination of the inside of her airway.

'I was thinking of scoping her next?' It was really a statement but I wanted confirmation my plan was the right one.

'Sounds good to me,' he agreed.

I handed over the patient's face mask and with it, control of her airway and anaesthesia to my consultant and picked up the long thin black fibre optic scope. Passing it through the nose, seeing my view on the monitor ahead I remembered all I'd been taught: follow the black hole, keep it in the middle of the screen, stay away from the walls, see the way ahead before advancing the scope and pray not to cause any bleeding. The internal air space was severely narrowed, the tissues angry and inflamed, swollen to twice their usual size, encroaching upon it. The scope passed down behind the tongue. This time I could see the epiglottis. It was fat and thick and was blocking the pathway to the vocal cords. I deftly maneuvered the scope behind it and upwards. There was the V shaped opening I was looking for. I advanced slowly through the angry looking vocal cords to see the cartilaginous rings of the trachea. I continued on, hardly daring to breathe, until I saw the airway branch right and left at the carina. I was almost there. Tentatively, I began to pass the breathing tube over the telescope. I twisted it through the nose, ignoring the painful sounding crunch it made. I advanced it further down the scope, knowing I was going for broke. It was all or nothing now. I could see the cords opening and closing with respiration, swollen and restricted in their movement. I had forgotten to specify a smaller, more narrow tube to the nurse who had set up the equipment but it was too late to change it now. With a final anti-clockwise rotation the tube advanced through the narrowed opening and into the windpipe. I withdrew the scope, observing the tube remaining in the trachea. I fumbled to attach the breathing system and looked anxiously at the screen. After an agonising few seconds the first little white blip appeared on the carbon dioxide monitor. The exhaled gas not only a sign of life but of correct tube placement in the respiratory system.

'Bravo', the deep voice of my consultant boomed.

I managed to control my surprise at the praise *and* my shaking hands sufficiently to give the intravenous drugs into Kirsty's drip to deepen the anaesthetic and finally, relax the patient.

I exhaled, unaware I had been holding my breath. I felt exhausted. My arms ached from holding up the scope. My back and hamstrings ached from leaning over the head of the bed. But I was elated. I had succeeded in performing, under stress, the anaesthetic technique most feared by registrars. The patient was alive. I had saved the patient. I had long known what to do but now I knew I could actually do it, and in an extreme emergency. I could actually do it, and I had done it.

Time returned to normal speed at that point and conversation resumed in the theatre. Activity began to get the patient ready for transfer to intensive care. She would remain sedated until the swelling had resolved sufficiently to pose no further threat to her airway. At this time it would be safe to awaken the patient and remove the breathing tube.

When I returned to my on call room I was too wired to get back to sleep. I reflected on the events. I had spent five years at medical school, one year as a house officer, another year as a casualty doctor and seven years training as a specialist in anaesthesia. Next week I would begin my first Consultant job. Was I ready? Was I fit for purpose? I decided I probably was both of these things and that a long arduous journey had resulted in my arrival at the prized destination. For the first time, I felt reassured by my ability. My years of training had delivered and I was now ready to call myself a consultant. Looking back to the very beginning, I realised what a long way I had come.

2. My First Time

Rewind 12 years and I was about to enter an operating theatre for the first time. This occasion remains one of my worst experiences there.

It was the beginning of the third year at medical school, our first year in the hospital, meeting real patients. Prior to this we had spent two years learning a mass of human physiology, anatomy, and pharmacology; the components of normal structure and function of the human body. We learnt how its systems work when well and how they are altered by disease processes and affected by drugs we administer. Now it was time to see it all in action.

I was attached to a general surgical department along with five others. We were equally nervous, scared and excited, full of anticipation about finally arriving on the wards, learning to be doctors.

One day we split into two groups of three. One for the out patient clinic and the other to go to theatre with the surgical registrar. I was going to theatre!

I should mention that this was a big deal. Huge. The surgeon was loud, arrogant, male, and typically impatient but despite this there was something god-like about him. He was a proper doctor, that to which we aspired. Further, he was a surgeon! He could do operations on people! And we were about to witness this first hand.

After two years of anatomical dissection we were used to the gory aspect of cutting up body parts so the fear of fainting in theatre was somewhat diminished. The main worry was of making a fool of yourself, or being humiliated; questioned openly in front of the theatre team and not knowing the answer.

He dashed off in the direction of the theatre suite and we followed obediently behind.

The stress began immediately. He showed me the door to the female changing room where I was to change into scrubs and meet him in theatre. It sounded easy and oh so casual as he left taking the two boys with him to the male changing room. I did not know the code for the door. There was no one around so I knocked. Repeatedly. 'Hello?' I shouted, more than once. After a seemingly prolonged period of time the door was open by someone in full theatre garb. She glanced at my medical student identity badge and allowed me to enter. I took in the rows and rows of lockers, the jumble of footwear lying around and the piles of blue clothes. (Blue! I thought they would be green; everyone referred to them as 'greens' after all.)

Before she hurried off, I quickly asked for help.

'Excuse me, I've to get changed for Mr Benson's theatre?'

'Help yourself to clothes and try to find a matching pair of clogs. Hats over there by the sinks and masks in theatre. Don't leave anything valuable in here. When you're ready go it's out that door and turn left. He's in theatre 6' she explained, all this at 100 miles per hour as she carried on her way.

I was aware I was already late by having waited outside the door for so long and felt panicked. I looked at the piles of theatre clothes that filled an entire wall. No-one had told me that the colour coding of the trims equated with small, medium and large sizes so I tried on a few, hurriedly discounting the tiny ones and the huge ones, desperately hoping no one would come in and catch me returning them untidily to the shelf. Eventually I donned a pair that fitted, in the broadest sense of the word. (Theatre clothes are generally referred to as 'each size fits no-one', but I was blissfully unaware of that at the time.)

Next, shoes. There was a box of shoes, but each had a name written on the heel. Would I be in trouble if I borrowed someone else's shoes? Could I assume that person was not at work if their plastic clogs were in the box? Did they simply share shoes here? I shuddered at the thought! What else could I do? The smell of sweaty feet from the box was pungent and the plastic clogs were splashed and stained with various unknown fluids. Using my fingertips I picked through the box. I found several clogs in my size, but all for the left foot. Looking around I saw a matching pair lying on the floor close by. There was no size on them but they were only slightly too big and I decided they would do.

Right. Next, a hat. Over by the sinks there were four boxes of hats, all the girl style with wavy elastic rather than the more square, authoritative style with ties for the men. The hats came in four colours: blue, green, pink and white. The pink was too sickly sweet and white would make me look washed out. I chose blue because it would match the blue clothes and carefully arranged it so my fringe was still visible (was that allowed?) and I didn't look quite so idiotic. I breathed a sigh of relief that I was now, ready to go into theatre. I was subsequently to learn that blue hats were for doctors, pink for nurses, green for operating department practitioners (ODPs) and white for students from any discipline. Who knew? I wasn't a mind reader after all.

I found the door that led into the theatre suite and found theatre six. I put on a mask and timidly entered noting my male colleagues already there, looking relaxed and chatting to each other.

The patient was already anaesthetised. Sister had just finished setting up the instruments. My registrar was getting scrubbed up.

'Have a look at the veins now,' he yelled

Everyone turned to see who he was talking to and, feeling even more conspicuous, I approached the table. Was it okay to examine the patient? I asked the anaesthetist. She smiled and nodded 'go ahead'.

As I was about to begin examining the leg, Sister moved in closer to the operating table, holding up an iodine soaked sponge to begin to prepare the leg for surgery.

'Stand back! Out the way!' she said shortly.

I immediately took a step backwards, right into her trays of sterile instruments. I stumbled as I lost my balance, sending her trolley flying across the floor.

As the crash of falling metal instruments subsided, there was a pause, the calm before the storm and I held my breath.

Horror. Dismay. Embarrassment. Shame. I could not think of anything worse.

Again, everyone turned to look at me and I sensed they too, were holding their breath. Sister's eyes, visible between her hat and mask flashed with anger and bore into me. I wondered if perhaps looks really could kill?

'You. Have. Just. Contaminated. ALL the instruments!' she shouted at me.

Before I could think about responding, attention was quickly diverted from me as a small fierce looking woman burst into theatre leaving the swing door quivering in her wake. She too looked as if about to explode. (What was it about the women here I wondered?)

'Miss Brown! Hello. How can we help you?' Sister was most polite all of a sudden.

'My shoes are not where I left them in the changing room! I cannot imagine anyone daring to borrow them but when I find them...'

I didn't stop to ask if she meant finding the shoes or the person wearing them. Instead I scurried out of theatre, hopefully unnoticed, back to the changing room, to rid myself of the contraband shoes.

Could this day get any worse I wondered?

3. A Career Choice

As a medical student, although I had no idea which specialty of medicine I would choose to pursue for a long time, I was always fascinated by the brain. Not in a 'want to be a brain surgeon' kind of way though; neurosurgery combines the most hostile of surgeons with an awfully sad patient population: young adults with devastating head injuries and parents in their prime with life changing brain tumours.

No, I was amazed at the brain and its ability to function at such a high standard of complexity and knowledge. Continually adjusting and adapting to keep the body ticking over no matter what we threw at it. Fad diets, fasting, over eating, running a marathon, and boozing too frequently all present stress to the body and the brain sees this and sets in motion processes to balance out our aberrations and keep us alive, awake, functional and well. The more I learnt about the brain in those first two years of pure science at university, the more amazed I became.

As I discovered how the liver tightly controlled glucose metabolism, I couldn't help but think that my brain already knew this, it already does this, and is doing this for me right now! While studying for exams trying to remember how nerve endings met and transmitted their information to make muscles work or hormone levels change, I was frustrated that this knowledge was already in my brain somewhere, yet I could not access it nor transfer it to the 'exam revision storage area'.

When we began to study the gross anatomy of the brain I found it incredible that the bulky piece of grey, amorphous, rubbery stuff that looked nothing special was, in fact a complex mass of nerves. I imagined the microscope would show it as a structure similar to a bouncy ball made from elastic bands. Tangled within the bundle of nerves were contacts and connections, each with areas where tiny amounts of hormone and transmitters acted to produce and amplify profound effects. Utterly amazing.

I visited a psychic medium at the beginning of my fourth year at university, I'm not sure why as I, am scepticism personified. I like science and facts, not incense and crystals.There were a lot of airy fairy comments that I could trot out too, to anyone paying me fifty quid. Talk of 'challenges ahead', a need to 'persevere to succeed' and 'finding a special type of happiness'. Once she knew I was a medical student, she told me I would excel in psychiatry. (I assumed she meant as a doctor rather than one afflicted by psychiatric disease.) I didn't take her predictions too seriously as she also insisted I was involved in amateur dramatics and one day would hog the limelight centre stage! Nothing could be further from the truth in this regard, but I kept an open mind.

Having never considered a career in psychiatry before then, I wondered if it would be a specialty where I could study the actions of the brain and treat those with disease and illness of the brain manifesting itself in all sorts of different ways? I spent the next six months eagerly awaiting my psychiatry attachment, hoping to feel some sign that this was what I had been looking for, where I was destined to do great things, according to the wizened old fortune teller in the purple dress.

On the first day of the psychiatry attachment, we were told to observe the consultant interviewing a long term patient. The patient had kindly agreed to help us learn and would have the consultation in front of an audience of green, gaping, medical students.

She looked bizarre. She entered the room and eyed us with suspicion. I eyed her in amazement. She had a wide eyed, slightly crazed look and wild orange hair sticking out everywhere. She was adorned with lots of unusual, noisy jewellery and inflicted with the poorest dentition I had ever seen. She spoke slowly with a posh accent and described to us her flamboyant life. I had no idea what age she was.

She was well travelled, had lived in many different cultures, enjoyed music and indeed had written a few pieces that a national orchestra would be performing shortly. Her bracelets and bangles had been gifts from local tribes on the banks of the river Nile and she reminisced about her time spent there. Most of it sounded plausible, if slightly atypical. As the interview went on, I realised some of what she said was contradictory and other parts simply impossible: she had been 'gifted' a child by an African taxi driver. She was very unwell during the pregnancy and, believing this meant the baby was evil, she gave it up for adoption immediately after it was born. I was naive at the time and more than slightly surprised when near the end, we were shown the extent to which the whole story was a display of her illness. The consultant asked her to tell us her name and the date. Did she remember why we were present? Oh yes, she was the Queen of Sheeba, we were her followers and we had listened well during the last hour as she educated us. It was 1925.

The experience did not ignite any true interest in me, much less any passion. In fact, I was a bit puzzled. I was not entirely sure the patient believed what she was saying, not sure that she was truly *unwell*. She may just be pretending to be outrageous and shocking. Who knew? I could not believe what I could not see and quantify. The patient looked physically well and I could not 'see' how her brain was unwell, not in the way I could measure low blood pressure or find the heart beat irregular.

The whole episode was too far removed from reality, from normality, for me to comprehend and I eliminated psychiatry as a career choice, leaving it to join a worryingly long list of other specialities I had sampled and eliminated too.

I never considered surgery seriously. It was not for me, not a job I was cut out for (pardon the pun). Cutting bits out of patients in full view of the team requires an arrogance I do not possess, despite what some may believe.

I had no patience for general practice with its array of social problems and mountains of paperwork.

I was frustrated by the timescale in general hospital medicine where wise doctors would ponder and debate, show casing their advanced knowledge and preening their feathers, before increasing the dose of diuretic a smidgen and waiting a full week before re-checking the patient and blood tests.

Both these options seemed burdened by an ongoing duty of care to patients with chronic diseases who improved oh so slowly, if indeed at all. It was frustrating to watch patients take three steps forwards and two steps backwards. Nothing seemed to be complete, never finished. There was no definitive end point in the treatment process.They presented again and again. At times a little bit worse, others a little better.

Radiologists sat in dark rooms all day that I imagined to be cold and lonely, at risk of inducing hibernation. Ophthalmology was way too difficult; I had only ever pretended to visualise the back of the eye when handed the ophthalmoscope in clinic and never understood all the squiggly figures and measurements written in the notes.

However, when I reach final year at medical school, I had an inkling I may want to do anaesthesia even although this was largely by process of elimination. I was yet to experience the subject but I thought it would address the areas of dissatisfaction I had identified in other specialities. I thought it would meet my criteria for the perfect job. Put them to sleep, wake them up at the end, job done. No tinkering at the edges of treatment regimes, no hanging around waiting for the drugs to work. It would be fast, decisive and effective. A new day would bring new patients keeping it fresh and interesting. Above all, the anaesthetist always knew what to do! What not to like?

The first time I met a consultant anaesthetist was during a resuscitation training afternoon in my final year at medical school. She was called Dr Black and she was teaching us on a mannikin how to hold the face mask onto a patient's face to administer rescue breaths if found unconscious and not breathing (the patient, obviously.) She was full of joie de vivre and her enthusiasm was intoxicating. She was colourful, confident and loud while making the skills look easy. Above all she was inspiring and at the end of the session I decided I would take up her offer to attend one of her theatre sessions to gain some hands on experience of anaesthesia.

Several days later I left the ward during my medical placement and navigated my way through the changing rooms to find her theatre. My confidence surrounding theatre visits was much higher now that I had a defined purpose for going, a senior who was expecting me, and who would (hopefully) protect me from any nursing staff bullying or surgical banter at my expense. The case had just begun when I entered the theatre. I met Dr Black and reminded her of who I was. I was quickly learning to introduce myself to everyone at every juncture. Like any enthusiast, she was pleased to meet an interested student and launched forth about the current patient and his anaesthetic.

I was fascinated as she explained what was going on. The whoosh of the ventilator making the patients chest rise and fall, the steady blip blip blip tone of the heart monitor confirming the patient's well being, and a myriad of other tracings and monitors which enabled her to maintain a status quo within the patient as the operation proceeded. What I was not aware of that day, was her constant vigilance. While she chatted to me she appeared fully focussed on our conversation, keeping it at my level of knowledge. I now know she had half an eye on the carbon dioxide monitor, half an eye on the progress of the operation and an ear out for any change in the tone of the pulse probe, signifying a drop in the patient's oxygen level.

As the end of the operation neared, she gave the patient, what seemed like a little bit of this and that from several little syringes each with a colourful label with the names of drugs I'd never heard of printed on them. She showed me the switch that controlled the mechanical ventilator and flipped it, thus switching it off and transferring our attention to the green reservoir bag hanging from the breathing system, a length of plastic tubing emerging from the anaesthetic machine. We were to watch the bag for movement she said, which would begin as the patient started to breathe for himself again. The patient must re-establish their regular breathing pattern before we could turn off the anaesthetic gases and wake him up fully.

Several minutes passed and the bag did not move. Dr Black did not seem perturbed and the patient's oxygen level remained high. This amazed me. No breathing yet still alive and well? This was due to the storage in the lungs of additional oxygen given during the procedure now being utilised. This was physiology in action and I found it incredible.

Another doctor stuck his head around the door of theatre at that point and beckoned to Dr Black to come over to talk with him. With a final glance around our station she moved away, the whole six feet to the door away. I continued to watch the bag. I stared at it, willing it to move. I glanced over, she was still talking at the door but gave me a nod and a smile. Seconds passed. Then perhaps minutes. Who knew exactly? It felt like hours. The patient was not breathing. The bag was not moving. The ventilator was switched off and the chest was not going up and down. I began to worry and stared at the bag even harder, wondering if I saw a flicker of movement akin to the distant shimmer of water in the desert. There was none. As my anxiety grew, Dr Black continued her conversation, unaware of my discomfort. (Although 'rising panic' would describe my feelings more accurately). I wondered if she had forgotten I was only a medical student. Had her concentration been diverted from the patient with her conversation? I felt a burden of responsibility. The patient's life was literally hanging in the balance in front of me and I was standing, frozen to the spot, doing nothing to improve the situation. I knew I had to do something. I tried and failed to catch her eye again. Still no breathing. The bleeps continued at their steady rate and tone, in contrast to my mounting agitation.

'Dr Black? The patient's still not breathing! The bag has not moved!' The words were involuntary. I was surprised to hear them aloud and they seemed to come of their own volition.

She turned and glanced at the patient, the monitors, the bag, and at me. She looked not the slightest bit concerned.

'Give it a squeeze if you like then, that might get him going' she offered airily.

Me? Squeeze the bag? Squeeze life into the patient?

Suddenly I felt important. I felt useful. I felt the patient's life was truly in my hands. I had never felt like this before.

I kept my eye on his chest and reached for the green bag. Slowly I squeezed it, imagining the inflation bringing the patient back to life.

The green bag collapsed like a deflated balloon as I squeezed it, emptied it of gas and it remained in that flaccid state. Dormant. Empty. Squashed in my palm. Nothing happened. Had it worked? I could no longer tell if it was moving or not. The bleeps continued. Had they changed? Should I squeeze the bag again? But now there was nothing in it to squeeze. Where did the gas come from? Dr Black continued to chat. Did she think I was reliably delivering life-giving air to the patient? That I was breathing for him until he woke up? What if he died while I was doing nothing?

'Dr Black? Dr Black!' I called loudly, more desperately than the first time.

Now she turned and said the words to her companion that were music to my ears: 'I'd better go and get this lad off the table. Talk soon.'

With that she returned to my side and I felt my own heart rate begin to calm down. I was no longer in charge. It was not my responsibility.

Dr Black turned the valve above the green bag causing it to close and allowing it to fill with gas again. She gave it a couple of firm squeezes, saw the patient's chest rise and fall, and then waited. Within seconds the bag began to move itself. The patient's abdomen started to move up and down and mist formed in the breathing tube. He was breathing. All he had to do now was wake up! Fantastic! I was so excited you would be forgiven for thinking he had come back to life, but in some ways he had! He had started working again and it was amazing to witness for the first time.

Despite my panic that day I realised that anaesthesia at its most basic, is about keeping patients alive. Anything additional is a bonus. As long as the air goes in and out and the blood goes round and round, the worst that can happen is the patient wakes up which is by far preferable to them not waking up.

Anaesthesia was for me. It was fast, acute. It was life and death. I was sold.

4. Who is the Anaesthetist Anyway?

'So, not a proper doctor then?' was the disappointed response from a family friend when I confirmed I had chosen to specialise in anaesthesia. It had taken some time to convince my non medical family that I was truly staying in hospital medicine for good, that I would never be a general practitioner, everyone's idea of a real doctor. Explaining that I would be spending a further seven years of training to attain the status of hospital consultant in anaesthesia, seemed a further blow to them, compounding their disappointment that I hadn't quite 'made the grade'.

Despite being the largest of all hospital specialities and seeing more than 70% of all patients admitted to hospital, many people fail to realise that anaesthetists, in the United Kingdom, are actually doctors first and foremost. And who can blame them? Many members of the medical profession themselves don't know what we do (or why we do it) so how can we expect the public to know? (In the United States of America, the doctors are known as anesthesiologists and they oversee the work, much of it being done by nurse anaesthetists. See? Confusing.)

Recognising that the anaesthetist is a doctor is not as easy as it may appear. Many anaesthetic doctors arrive at work in scruffy jeans and jumpers and immediately change into theatre scrubs or 'blues'. Some introduce themselves to patients saying only 'Hi I'm Jane, I'm going to knock you off to sleep today' which does nothing to infer that Jane is a highly trained professional about to take responsibility for your life.

In my career to date, as an anaesthetist I have been mistaken for a porter and a cleaner and I am regularly asked by patients when the doctor will be along to see them. It is clear to me that many people do not know who or what the anaesthetist is so before I go any further I will clarify this.

Anaesthetists provide anaesthesia for each surgical speciality. In addition we run the intensive care unit 24 hours a day 7 days a week, we have a constant presence on the labour ward and see patients in the pain management clinic for chronic, intractable or terminal pain from any cause.

Most patients will have seen an anaesthetist for one reason or another, although they may not realise this at the time and almost certainly will not remember us afterwards.

General anaesthesia, being 'knocked out' or 'put under' remains a mystery. The mechanism of action of general anaesthetics on the brain and central nervous system are not fully understood, yet their efficacy remains high and reliable throughout the population. Patients are forgiven for thinking once the needle is in the back of their hand, the job is pretty much done until the end of the operation when they will miraculously awaken, just at the right time. This apparent simplicity can and does occur in many operations, and is judiciously controlled by the anaesthetist. When anaesthesia is carried out well, it looks terribly simple but when devoid of skill, precision and timing, this can change in a flash and it looks simply terrible.

Few realise that ten seconds after that little injection in the back of the hand it is routine for the airway to obstruct as it relaxes. That passage from the mouth and nose down to the lungs, which is vital for life, needs to be propped open and supported by someone or something immediately.

Nor is it known that spontaneous breathing stops as consciousness is lost. If ventilation is to continue it must be taken over by the anaesthetist squeezing a bag of air into the lungs or delegating this job to a mechanical ventilator. Finally the side effects of the drugs: plummeting blood pressure and s-l-o-w-ing of the heart rate as you drift off to sleep need to be monitored, diagnosed and immediately corrected. Pain relief for each procedure is planned and administered. The reflex actions and reactions of the human body to the stress of a surgical operation are anticipated and actively managed to maintain the patient's status quo. All in all it is a lot more than a little jab in the back of the hand, but then I would say that of course.

So, I *am* a proper doctor, but I'm not a GP. There is no 'yet'.

It is common for well educated members of the public, and even surgeons, to wonder what we actually *do* during the operation. After inducing general anaesthesia with the big syringe and stabilising the patient with the little syringe, boring old anaesthesia seems a strange choice of career when compared to the excitement of surgery, the glamour of accident and emergency or the intellectual prestige of hospital medicine. As a junior house officer straight from medical school, my first boss, a consultant physician looked at me with horror when I stated my intention was to pursue a career in anaesthesia. 'What a waste.' he said, '*You* could make it as a physician, you know.'

The truth is I enjoy the only vague understanding of our role and I love to maintain the mystery, play down the importance and seem surprised when anyone suggests it may be a tad mundane.

Indeed, on pre-operative visits, patients often make suggestions to help me deal with this period of complacency and potential boredom which I may suffer as their surgery is carried out. They can even sound slightly guilty as if they are holding me up, making me wait until the very end of the operation.

After explaining to one patient that her operation may take several hours, she offered me her suduko puzzle book to keep me occupied while she was asleep. As an afterthought she said I could also have her bag of Wether's Originals as I would probably miss my lunch and besides, she was fasting.

Other well-meaning patients have offered me their newspapers or magazines to fill the intra-operative void and one asked if there was a pay-as-you-go television in theatre as well as in the wards. If so I could watch 'Murder she wrote' during the afternoon session he suggested. I'm sure there was no pun intended.

At least these patients assumed I would be hanging around after the jab in the back of the hand.

I have been asked by another patient how I would know when to come back to wake her up. Would the surgeon have his secretary call me to let me know he was closing up? Or would I pop my head back into theatre every so often to see how he was getting on? What if I was at the canteen when the operation neared completion? No, I reassured her, I would be there all the time.

Another time, I was pleasantly surprised when an older gentleman asked me to explain what I would be doing while he was asleep.

I launched enthusiastically into my spiel about monitoring vital signs, making adjustments to the anaesthetic, balancing the level of pain relief with the degree of surgical stimulation, providing hydration and actively ensuring his temperature remained normal, liaising with the surgeon and so on.

'So you actually stay with me and look after me the whole time I'm under the anaesthetic?' he asked, eyebrows raised.

'Yes, that's correct,' I was pleased he seemed particularly insightful to the importance of my continued presence in theatre to his on-going welfare.

'Really?' he said, eyes now wide. 'That must be such an interesting job you have, imagine, getting to watch operations all day long'.

For once I did not know what to say. Yes, anaesthesia may appear boring but that means it is smooth, uncomplicated, routine and anaesthetists like that. This is our 'plan A' and it means it is being followed. Life would be too stressful if each anaesthetic was a hair-raising roller coaster of crisis management and near misses resulting in our own heart rate being higher than the patient's. It would also prevent us sitting back to write our chart neatly with a pretty pen and of course, admire the surgery.

5. Why Become an Anaesthetist?

Doctors are attracted to Anaesthesia, Intensive Care and Pain management (to give the specialty it's fully evolved title) for a variety of reasons. Some are technical geeks who always wanted to be Inspector Gadget when they grew up and now continue to be fascinated by machines, monitors, gas flows, pressure waves, bleeping noises and transducers, not to mention the joy of taking things apart to 'see how they work.'

Others like the solitude; the ability to work alone, not having too much interaction with the awake patient. The relative freedom from any continuity of care after the peri-operative period is enjoyed by many anaesthetists, in contrast to the surgeons.

However, there is no 'team' of anaesthetists. There is no entourage of ranked individuals visiting the wards, doing their rounds each morning where the great leader orates uninterrupted and the junior most underling scribbles it all down in the notes and on his (or her) 'to do' list. Processions like these are the reserve of surgeons and physicians. In anaesthesia we work alone the majority of the time. Our visits to the wards are practical and informative, and proceed without any great fuss after we have found the notes, accessed the blood results and found a spare terminal to log onto the e-prescribing system and identify the drugs the patient normally takes. No hassle at all!.

Quiet, often introverted individuals, while suited to anaesthesia, can be at great risk of mental illness and suicidal tendencies. They are drawn to the specialty which tolerates these traits but one that also provides access to potent, dangerous, controlled drugs that can be used, abused and can hasten death. I wonder if this is the sub-conscious reasoning of some who drift into the specialty.

Others say they enjoy the speed of anaesthesia. You may be surprised there is speed involved in anaesthesia as we are usually depicted on television doing very little during an operation, other than looking bored or doing the crossword perhaps, awaiting further instruction from the surgeon. This is not so. Potent drugs given intravenously cause rapid loss of consciousness and cessation of breathing in well patients who were, only moments before, walking, talking, and breathing. Inducing anaesthesia is an active, exciting display of acute pharmacology and physiology with a background frisson of potential danger. Rarely is more than

15 seconds spent waiting for the drugs to work, before more is given or another is added to the mix. Man meets medicine and the two interact in a myriad of ways, some helpful and intended, less so. Some predictable and not quite so helpful and others coming completely out of the blue causing an untold degree of mayhem.

Role models are an important factor in determining anyone's career choice. Looking up to someone senior to you, who is respected and in control can be intensely motivating, particularly when they exhibit skills you do not yet possess. The most experienced anaesthetists have an ability to bring a seemingly chaotic situation efficiently into one of calm and control with a methodical and planned approach. At times the mere presence, or arrival of a senior has this type of calming, reassuring effect on a stressful situation before they have contributed anything practicable.

After my junior doctor year I wanted some more experience of doctoring before heading to the mysterious world of anaesthesia so I spent a year working in Accident and Emergency as it was called at the time. It is now called the department of Emergency Medicine and in between times it has been called a variety of others things too, amongst which feature 'casualty' or the insulting yet humorous 'department of casual medicine'. It's name is beside the point. In this year, my desire to train in anaesthesia was confirmed.

I longed for the day I could attend to one patient at a time, giving them my full attention and planning subsequent patients to follow; the work rate determined largely by the surgeon and out of my hands. In casualty however, as it became busier we each had to work faster and spread ourselves thinner. Times when patients waited in radiology for an x-ray or waited for their blood results from the lab was time when we squeezed in another one or two new patients and ended up working as hairdressers do, fitting in clients for quick cuts between those waiting for their hair colour to 'take'. It was exhausting, confusing and easy to get mixed up and make mistakes.

Your reputation in casualty is defined by your performance in 'resus'; the resuscitation room at the back door where the 999 ambulances deliver the sickest patients directly. These are live or die moments for the patient as well as your on-going six month contract. The ambulances called in ahead on a dedicated line to our red, flashing, light up bat phone. Everything would pause as we observed the charge nurse answer the call. I would spend the next few minutes before its arrival scanning every junior doctor's bible; the 'cheese and onion'.

Every junior doctor owns a copy a little green and yellow book called 'The Oxford

Handbook of Clinical Medicine'. It is widely known as the 'cheese and onion' reflecting its publication at a time now past when cheese and onion flavoured crisps *always* came in a green and yellow bag, regardless of their brand. This book is a must have for all newly qualified doctors and fit snugly in the deep pockets of our white coats (back in the days when we wore white coats and they were cleaned and starched by the hospital laundry).

Cheese and onion lists one medical condition per page and describes the diagnostic and management steps you should take for each one, and crucially, suggests when you should ask for specialised help. It gave us permission to ask for help. It also has a page on each and every medical emergency that you may be presented with. These pages have red tops so you can find them in a hurry with trembling hands before the ambulance drivers burst through the doors with the stretchered patient. This frequently consulted chapter on (how to deal with terrifying) 'Medical emergencies' gives a step by step approach to managing life threatening conditions such as severe asthma, prolonged seizures and coma. The scary first line on each page is an alert 'Fast action saves lives' emblazoned across the top. This is followed by 'A calm atmosphere helps the patient' at the beginning of the treatment section (it also helps the doctor I would add) and the very last line, squeezed onto the bottom of every page was 'If still no improvement, call the anaesthetist'.

Basically, if the treatment outlined on the page has not improved the patient's condition and the proverbial is hitting the fan, call the anaesthetist to sort it out for you. This is because the anaesthetist always knows what to do in an emergency and I figured that by becoming an anaesthetist, I too, could transcend upon chaotic scenes with a zen-like calm, soothing the frayed edges while quietly transforming the situation into a state of control and stability.

After the stress of managing a breathless patient, an unconscious patient or a fitting patient, the resplendent sight of the anaesthetic registrar in a shining armour of blue, distinguished by a hat and a stethoscope worn casually around their neck, brought intense relief. They would be forgiven for their 'Arrive, Blame and Criticise' approach to the A,B,C of emergencies and we would hurry to fulfill their every request. Everything was going to be okay now they were here and we bent over backwards to keep them happy. They would administer some drugs into the arm, sending the patient off to sleep and bringing their distress to an end. A state of calm would prevail as they opened the mouth and inserted a tube into the patients windpipe to allow their breathing to be assisted and monitored. Next, without batting an eyelid, they would insert a further large intravenous drip into the hand in which we had struggled even to see a vein, never mind cannulate one.

Once stabilised and packaged up securely, the anaesthetist would take the patient away to theatre or intensive care. They would exit our resuscitation room, a distinguished procession moving slowly, monitors bleeping, ignoring the passing visitors who stopped and stared, as they concentrated on their lap of honour towards the corridor.

The anaesthetists and their assistants appear humble, accepting of our respect, while basking in the knowledge that they have saved the day for us. We indulge them and allow them this moment of celebrity, for glory is scarce as an anaesthetist. Their great achievements in the operating theatre are expected and rarely commented upon. Their value is not visible. Anaesthesia does not cure illness and disease and leaves no neat scar. The bottle of whisky and tickets to the corporate box are reserved for surgeons and cardiologists who perform visible, perceivable miracles.

For the reasons mentioned, the anaesthetic registrar is the most highly regarded doctor on call in the hospital overnight. Senior enough to have a few years training and experience under their belts yet junior enough to be manning the frontline on site and therefore be immediately available. This is who you will call to get you out of trouble. This is who will take over when you are out of your comfort zone and the chips are down. Anaesthetists have a set of skills which makes it incredibly difficult for anyone to die whilst they are present. This is not arrogance. This is the reality of what they are trained to do, manage critical illnesses. Many a junior doctor has dawdled out of his or her on call room to attend the cardiac arrest call to ensure the anaesthetist will arrive ahead of him, take charge, and get things moving in the right direction. I know this because I have been that doctor.

The paradox is that when fully trained, consultant anaesthetists fall firmly at the lower end of the medical hierarchy. If you want the glory do not enter anaesthesia. If you want public displays of affection from grateful patients, don't do anaesthesia. If you want professional respect from other consultants, don't do anaesthesia. Orthopaedic surgery, cardiology and acute medicine are much better choices for each of these aspirations respectively.

To go right back to the start, it was 1997 and I had secured a novice anaesthetic training post. A two year contract, subject to review every six months and renewable if appropriate progress was being made. I was elated, but already felt under immense pressure to perform, to meet the standards expected, as my career got underway.

6. The First Day

On my first day of anaesthetic training I turned up a mixture of nerves and excitement. There were three of us and we were met by one of the awesome registrars previously mentioned. He gave us a tour of the department, the expensive scare unit (his own clever name for the intensive care unit) and onto the theatre suite. He gave us lots of information and it was impossible to take much of it in. However he shared his three rules by which we should abide if we were to succeed in anaesthesia. These I did remember and they did indeed turn out to be true.

'Firstly, always remember you work *with* the surgeons and not *for* the surgeons. Secondly, beware of the bottom abscess and stand up to the surgeons.'

Patients with bottom abscesses are slipped onto the end of the list as 'just a small quick case' and typically come to theatre around midnight with a junior anaesthetist and an eager surgeon, keen to practice out of hours and out of sight of his boss. These patients are regularly challenging for the anaesthetist, the condition being associated with obese, hirsute, sweaty lorry drivers often sporting a ginger beard. Believe me when I say all these factors are pertinent and the 'simple surgical case' to which you have been talked into anaesthetising is actually a procedure fraught with problems and opportunity for disaster. Being a shy retiring wall flower is no way to deal with demands from a typical surgeon: a healthy degree of assertiveness is required from day one.

Thirdly, to address the fear most junior anaesthetists have of inadvertently killing a patient with anaesthesia when they have come in only for varicose vein surgery, he said to 'remember that as long as the air continues to go in and out, and the blood goes round and round, the worst that can happen is the patient wakes up'.

While this may sound like a disastrous outcome (and admittedly it is one of the worst things that can happen to a patient), when the alternative is death you would choose this option every time. Aware or dead? No brainer. This was a reassuring message. It was simple. While there was a huge amount we did not know and even more that we did not know that we did not know, this we did know. We *could* keep the air going in and out and the blood going round and round and sustain life. The bottom line in anaesthesia is that the patients are alive and awake before we begin, during the operation they are alive and asleep, and at the end of the operation they remain alive and are once again awake. The common word throughout is 'alive'. While awareness under anaesthesia is a tragic, but thankfully rare occurrence, death due to anaesthesia is inexcusable and irreversible.

The day was exhausting. I went home mentally and physically drained, my brain in a muddle and unsure how to sort itself out. Should I concentrate on learning the new drugs first? Or the new equipment or the new techniques? It was safe to say I was truly over-whelmed and did not know where to begin addressing this.

7. Getting Started

For the first few weeks new anaesthetists are always doubled up with a consultant for theatre sessions during day time hours. We are not allocated to any out of hours work until we have mastered the basics and are deemed capable and competent to be on call.

Being doubled up all the the time with no on call sounds like a dream job, devoid of responsibility, but the reality was very different.

The reality was five long days in a new environment, learning new skills that looked so easy but were nothing of the sort! I felt adrift at sea without navigation as I changed from being a competent relatively independent casualty doctor, to a complete novice in anaesthesia who did not know where to start and must not be left alone with an asleep patient.

The days were long and I quickly learnt the anaesthetists start before the surgeons and finish afterwards when they take last patient to recovery. The surgeons have breaks between the patients on the list but we cannot. We are required to keep things moving by waking the current patient up and getting the following one off to sleep efficiently and ready for surgery. Tea breaks for us are during the cases. (Well they are for me anyway, our consultants do not leave us alone even for a coffee break, instead they ask us to bring them one back with us.)

After the last patient is safely deposited in recovery, we find our list for the next day and trudge upstairs to the ward to see these patients pre-operatively.

The fatigue in those first few weeks is immense and I was surprised by this. I'm not sure whether it is due to mental exhaustion of continually learning and the stress of feeling useless, worrying about doing everything wrong even inadvertently or, if it was because, as rumour has it, we were not yet accustomed to breathing the anaesthetic gases which escape into the air and surround us.

During those early days in theatre we learnt how to put patients to sleep. Which drugs to use, how much to give, how quickly to give it and how to tell they were asleep because for such an important detail, there is no water tight sign, test, or monitor to confirm the patient is indeed adequately anaesthetised. We learned how to use a laryngoscope, the big metal blade to move the tongue aside allowing visualisation of the vocal cords. This ensured accurate placement of the breathing tube. We practiced what to do if this was unsuccessful: manually ventilating patients using a face mask and a self inflating bag until they woke up safely. These are the nuts and bolts of general anaesthesia. We learnt more about effective pain relief for operations and how to manage the expected negative effects of both surgery and anaesthesia on the body: the heart suddenly slowing, the blood pressure either surging or disappearing, the bleeding continuing, and gradually we became confident and able to anticipate and manage these problems reliably.

The first big step was being left alone in theatre while the consultant went to the coffee room. This was the beginning of our reins being loosened, the aim being to get us flying solo, covering the on call rota as quickly as possible.

Dr Roberts was one of the consultants I spent a lot of time with in theatres as he was one of the main trainers for the newbies. The first time he left me alone while he went for a coffee he pushed the soft comfy chair on wheels towards me. 'Here, you can have The Chair of Anaesthesia'. He said he would be 20 minutes and to call him back if I was worried.

I was worried the moment he left. Anything could happen in an instant. I found myself unable to sit down and was aware of tension in my neck and shoulders, I was clenching my jaw and found myself acting as if by keeping as still as possible this would prevent the patient moving and the nice steady state would remain unchanged!

I watched the monitors intently, listening to the bleeps and praying for nothing to happen until the boss was back. I looked at the surgeon. He seemed oblivious that the new apprentice was now alone at the helm, and I prayed he would not ask me to do anything, while the boss was away. What if I didn't hear him? What if I didn't know what he was saying from behind his mask?

I jumped as an alarm sounded. The heart rate had increased. A little. Did that matter? Should I do something about it? Now? Should I wait and see?

I looked at our little tray of drugs. Did I need to give any? The problem was not the actual giving of them into the drip, it was *deciding* to do so knowing that along with any benefit gained, there may be less desirable knock on effects that would upset the precarious status quo of the patient. I was terrified I would make things worse. Terrified I would be shouted at if I did the wrong thing.

'What do you want up next?' My mounting anxiety was broken by the ODP indicating the empty bag of intravenous fluid. Caught between two puzzles I struggled to make any decision.

'Err, emm,' I paused. The answer was a simple one but at that moment in my mind I was weighing up the fluids I knew of, trying to anticipate what Dr Roberts would want to use next, and whether the patient in fact needed more fluid: a full distended bladder is as undesirable during surgery as it is any other time. I didn't know the correct answer.

'Just the same again please' I tried to smile but my mouth was dry and my lips stuck to my teeth. I was aware I sounded more as if I was in the pub rather than running an anaesthetic.

'How fast do you want it going?'

'Not too fast, but not too slow either.' I replied hedging my bets.

The ODP had no doubt seen countless trainees in my position and I wondered if he was amusing himself at my expense as he set the drip to mid-speed.

As the weeks passed I became better at making the small decisions and carrying out the basic skills. As I improved, my supervision was weaned gradually, being moved further and further away over the following months. First to the recovery bay, then to the coffee room and later to the distant anaesthetic office, before eventually being left to fly solo with a consultant at home on the end of the telephone. At the same time I was being given more responsibility during the course of a procedure. I was left alone first of all to wake a patient up, then I was left alone to put another off to sleep. Just like a baby beginning to walk, I was enjoying my progress and excited by my rising competence and confidence, always ready for the next stage. However, it was several months before I relaxed enough to sit down during an operation.

8. Going On Call

The next stage of training included being on call, with out of hours duties. This meant having to provide anaesthesia for emergency operations that could not wait until the morning. If I needed help, there was a senior registrar on call who would discuss cases and advise us, or attend to help if required. There were three of us on call at any one time in my first hospital. We each covered a specific area of the hospital. One for intensive care, one for the labour ward and the most junior of them all was for theatres, and that was me. My extreme anxiety about this step up was made worthwhile by the badge of honour of actually being *the* anaesthetist on call: somebody somewhere thought I was up to the job even if my self belief was lacking.

The first night on call I barely slept. This was in part due to the on call room being next door to the hospital laundry which ran all night creating excessive heat and continual noise. The bed was also unfamiliar. The thin lumpy mattress was ancient; stained, frayed at the edges with bits of foam escaping. There were no windows in the room, it was more a large cupboard than a bedroom, yet comically, there was a small pelmet running along the top of one wall. I later learnt this was there to meet a ruling about the standard of furnishings required in on call rooms nationwide. One requirement was that rooms *must* have curtains. And indeed we had a curtain! So that was fine. What we were lacking was a window, but there was no such rule about windows, someone clearly assumed there would always be a window in a room without the need to mention it specifically. They forgot the golden rule; never assume anything. It's quite amazing how horrid rooms can meet the criteria and standards required, yet still be completely inadequate. It was almost funny.

The real problem preventing sleep was not the room or the bed. Going to sleep is associated with relaxation and security, feeling snug, feeling sleepy, looking forwards to closing your eyes and resting. Not one of these feelings were present when I began on call duties. As a junior I would eye my bleep suspiciously. Was it going to go off? Had the batteries gone flat? Would I miss a call if I had a shower? What would the call be for? Would I kill the patient? Would the registrar be angry if I called them? So many questions. So many anxieties.

I would lie in the lumpy bed when there was no work, wearing theatre blues as pyjamas, to be ready to run. Should I take my bra off I wondered? Very uncomfortable to sleep with it on, but what if I forgot to put it back on when called? Would I stop to brush my hair? No, wearing a hat in theatre meant messy hair was not an issue. Would I brush my teeth first? That takes a few minutes but I didn't want to breathe morning breath onto everyone else.

With my mind full of so many unknowns I lay awake watching the clock, seeing each hour pass so slowly. Usually, if I wake up at 3am I think 'excellent, four more hours to sleep' but when on call it's more a case of '3am? Is that all? Still another four hours during which anything can happen.' I wished the night would pass more quickly than it ever did. I looked forward to morning when my time became my own once more.

On the nights we were busy, I began to enjoy it. I felt important, responsible and entrusted to get on with a job alone. I watched my friends training to be surgeons, only being able to place a couple of skin sutures at the end of the operation. They were there with at least one if not two seniors. They did not know what operation was required until the abdomen was open. Would it be one they knew about? One they had seen before? What if it required a technique they had not yet learnt? In contrast I was alone with my ODP assistant. I could manage the whole process from beginning to end without my boss. I could give one safe, basic anaesthetic that would cover a multitude of surgical procedures. I enjoyed that independence early on in training.

There were some aspects I missed. Surgeons and physicians are a team and hunt in pairs, especially on call. They operate together, review patients together and go for dinner together. I was not part of a team. I was the lone anaesthetist for theatres. My colleagues were in remote areas of the hospital and often busy when I was not. My senior was at home and would only come in if necessary, not merely to keep me company. At times we did manage to meet in the department for a cup of coffee or in the canteen if we were lucky enough to be quiet during the few hours the hospital canteen remained open. (The numbers 8080 flashing on your pager, was a message from a colleague signalling they had 'ate nothing' and to meet them in the canteen.) But often this was not possible.

The theatre staff were a team. They had a history together and knew each other well (unlike the transient population of trainee doctors just passing through). They were usually doing their knitting, chatting or snoozing in the coffee room. So as well as being alone, on call is often lonely and this either suits you or it doesn't. Usually this doesn't bother me too much and I made use of my free time by reading magazines or watching television (if the coat hanger was angled correctly to allow reception) but always with the feeling that whatever I did, it would be far preferable to be doing it in the comfort of my own home. The hospital is not a homely place to spend the weekend.

The time I felt most alone (and sorry for myself) was at 5pm on Fridays when I was on call that night. It hit me hardest when I had progressed from covering theatre to working on an exceedingly busy, ten bedded intensive care unit.

In any intensive care unit you will find the sickest patients in the hospital. They usually have two or more systems failing in their body as a result of disease or injury. Most, but not all, are sedated with their breathing controlled by ventilators and although sicker, these patients are far easier to look after than the awake less unwell ones who pull out their drips and continually move around causing their monitors to alarm.

During the second year of training I felt a huge weight of responsibility descend upon me as I began overnight on calls for intensive care. As such, I would cover any eventualities on the unit but was also the first (or last, depending on how you look at it) port of call for other departments in the hospital. This included the emergency department and the resuscitation room. This was the place where I had first been impressed and inspired by anaesthetists and their ability to manage. Yet now I felt foolish and naive, an imposter with nowhere near the level of competence and ability to cope that I remember witnessing when I had been a junior in that department. Now I was terrified. Anything, absolutely anything could crash through the double doors from the ambulance bay and I would be required to deal with it. I tried to calm myself, remembering I could only deal with one patient at a time and that someone in my department thought me capable of working at this level. Before my first night on call for intensive care, I conjured up the words my mother would say. I could only do my best.

Most evenings you could hear the quiet whooshing of ventilators at each bed space after the relatives had left and the hustle and bustle of the day died down. The nurses would work quietly with their individual patients. A continual low murmur could be heard as they spoke to the unconscious patients while carrying out their duties aware that hearing often persists despite heavy sedation. The regular sounds of intensive care can be comforting and peaceful, but can also make you feel alone, as if in a ghost town no longer inhabited by real people.

It was worst on Fridays. Usually I love Fridays, but not when on call. Throughout the day I could sense the anticipation of the imminent weekend. Some outlined their social plans and boasted about the run of days off they had. Others showed a potent mix of motivation, frivolity and impending freedom. They would plough through their work to get it all done in time to float out of the hospital and begin their weekend plans on time. Meanwhile, I remained at work on Friday night, through until Saturday morning. I had the rest of Saturday off before being back on call for 24 hours on Sunday, finishing on Monday morning and back to day time work on Tuesday, to look forwards to.

This night, the unit was full. There were no spare beds. I learnt it is not the physical beds that are in short supply, nor the bed spaces that people talk of. The problem is one of money and staffing. If a unit is funded for five beds then it only has money to pay for round the clock staffing of five beds. Intensive care aspires to being a service rather than a location so if additional intensive care is needed most can stretch to five plus one patients and beds, for a short period at least. This is not the same as six beds; they are not funded for a 6th bed nor a 6th patient but squeezing another in, coping and managing, is easier than the alternative of transferring a patient to another hospital which is fraught with logistical difficulty.

As I waved everyone off, I received a call from the renal unit. They asked me to insert a central line into the neck of one of their patients who had 'difficult veins'. I groaned inwardly wondering if I should answer such calls with a friendly 'Dominos Venous Access Services', what would you like?'

The place suddenly seemed calm and quiet. The excitement of 5pm had come and gone and now we hunkered down to deal with the long night ahead. It reminded me of the one and only marathon I had run: great noise, excitement, and buoyancy at the starting point which fades after the first mile leaving you to get on with the mammoth task of the remaining 25 miles.

I had brought various books with me as I was studying for one of the exams. It is a funny idea to take books with you to work. The theory is good, if it is quiet you can study during working hours and not waste your own precious time doing it at home. In reality, it is preferable to be busy on call than to be quiet with no excuse not to study; the thought of studying only compounds the misery of working weekends and evenings when everyone else is having fun. Then there is the reverse psychology from the law of the sod, which states that the more books you bring to work, the busier you will be. The opposite is also true, when you have brought nothing to do you can almost guarantee a quiet on call.

In practice I never, ever studied whilst on call. At quiet times I would reason that, had I been busy, I would not have been able to study anyway so I should not feel too bad about being lazy and feeling disinclined to open a book.

Presumably I thought there was some kind of study god in the sky keeping track of how much I studied that I felt I had to justify my time in this way! No, on call was a time to be kind to yourself and this kindness often involved chips from the canteen, cake from intensive care and chocolate biscuits from the labour ward. Failing those options there was always vending machines for pure unadulterated chocolate and if you were lucky they would be in working order and not completely empty following the evening visiting hours.

Very quickly on Friday evenings the 'Crackerjack referrals' begin. Crackerjack was a childrens' television programme in my era and began with an overly loud announcement 'It's Friday! It's 5pm! It's Crackerjack!'

Crackerjack referrals to intensive care come at that very same time of the week when clinicians around the hospital realise they have unwell patients who may run into problems over the weekend. It suits them quite nicely if these patients are shipped to intensive care where any problems can be picked up and dealt with swiftly, saving them being called in from home. It was annoying on many grounds: the transparency of the request, the lack of planning and the practical time consuming aspect of reviewing a patient, deeming them unsuitable for intensive care and then justifying that decision to your own consultant, the referring consultant and often to the relatives who have been told prematurely their loved ones are moving to be observed more closely. You then become the bad doctor refusing to help their relative in contrast to their own good doctor who is trying to make it happen.

It is much quicker to admit patients to intensive care than it is to refuse admission with all the discussions it involves with nurses, patient, relatives and consultants. Sometimes I wonder if anyone is allowed to die in hospital anymore *without* being referred to intensive care to see if there is anything we can do. Only when it is pointed out that the patient has no reversible aspects to their illness and we are out of miracles right now, can their teams feel confident to allow nature to take its course.

Anyway, this evening the second referral came from the accident and emergency department. They had a young lad with an ecstasy overdose and could I please attend immediately.

This was interesting and I was down in flash. Central lines for renal patients can always wait. This could not. I had never seen an overdose or an aberrant reaction to ecstasy before although I knew of the fundamental problem of over heating and thirst.

I admit I was buzzing all of a sudden. As I entered the emergency department I took in the atmosphere. It was going like a fair, the noise level raised and commands and requests regarding this young man's treatment conveyed an air of urgency. Working alongside the casualty doctor, we each dragged up what we knew about the treatment, we consulted the cheese and onion of anaesthesia and phoned the poisons centre for advice and the rest of the management plan.

The patient was Tom and he looked younger than his 19 years. I introduced myself to him, more for his mother's benefit, as he continued to throw up into the cardboard bowls. His temperature was 40 degrees Celsius (over 100 fahrenheit) and the sweat was lashing off him. He smelled unpleasant. His talking was barely coherent and whatever his intention had been, it did not look much fun at this moment. His blood pressure was soaring, in part due to ecstasy and also from the effort of vomiting. His heart raced and was irregular at times as we raced to bring his temperature down and prevent a seizure. His mother stood staring, her face a mixture of concern, anger and fear. She was neatly dressed and looked normal really. Uncomprehending, as if dazed, she repeated that he'd never done anything like this before.

To actively cool him he was stripped. His t-shirt, cut off to avoid disturbing the vomit bowl and the monitors, looked forlorn as it lay in rags, much less adamant in it's anti-establishment slogan. We placed ice packs in his arm pits and groins, and a catheter into his bladder down which we instilled cold water and flushed it out again when warm, repeatedly. Usually we would use cold fluids intravenously but there is a danger of over-hydration and dangerous dilution of salts in the blood. There is no direct antidote to ecstasy but we furiously mixed up the thick orange powder of a notoriously insoluble drug, which helps to stabilise the abnormal cellular reaction which has been triggered.

I felt alive, purposeful, helpful and in control. I felt I was making a difference. After 90 minutes of treatment, the patient's temperature was remaining within the normal range. I secured his trolley and attached the portable monitoring ready for my lap of honour out of the resuscitation room up to intensive care.

This was why I chose anaesthesia. The poor referrals, the lack of beds, the calls for lines and the depression of 5 o'clock were forgotten for the time being.

9. Wrong Side Surgery

Whilst still a relatively junior trainee, I was allocated to regular 'solo lists'. This meant I was the only anaesthetist for a whole list of, usually minor, surgical procedures requiring general anaesthesia. The responsibility was mine alone.

As well as providing a service, working alone allowed us to practice our skills. It provided an opportunity to plan and run a list without a boss present to make subtle changes, to influence even the smallest decision and overrule any we made if he felt it necessary to do so. In essence, solo lists allowed us to try out what we were learning, make our own mistakes and learn how to sort them out. This is a highly effective way of making incidents memorable and deters us from repeating them in the future. Much of my practice remains based on events which occurred during my early solo lists, not all of them positive or planned.

The first time I had a solo list I was overcome with awe at the responsibility bestowed upon me. There it was in black and white, a formal theatre list typed up and displayed on the wall, on the wards, in the control desk folder.

SURGEON: Mr Sandhu
ANAESTHETIST: Dr May

I was buoyed by seeing my name in this way but simultaneously terrified. It was up to me, little old me, to get these patients off to sleep for their operations and to awaken them safely when complete. Only me! Somebody obviously thought I had the ability to do this. I only wished I felt as sure. So much could go wrong, there are so many junctures where a tiny deviation from the expected can have significant consequences. It was best not to dwell too much on what *may* or may not happen. It was much better to focus on the job in hand, focus on the fact that I had done this many times before, and usually it all goes to plan and nothing bad happens. I tried to rest assured that I had learnt the emergency drills and that they were stored away in my mind, ready for activation and automation if required.

Once I got used to seeing the bold headline, I quite enjoyed seeing my name displayed in this manner and looked forward to my solo lists.

On the day of this mistake, I had four patients on my list, three for excision of lumps and bumps and another for removal of infected toenail.

This fourth patient was 12 years old and had learning difficulties. He was listed for removal of an ingrowing great toenail following recurrent infection. He had twice before absconded from the day ward before surgery, in fits of temper and hysteria. This time he had been brought into the ward early to have a 'heavy, sedative premed in advance,' it stated in the notes, to prevent a similar scenario happening a third time. Indeed his parents had been assured it would not occur a third time! No pressure then.

This was not the usual straight forward case I was used to taking on alone. Big children can be difficult and physically strong. Communication is difficult when learning difficulties are present and a lack of understanding can make these children non compliant. It was fair to say I was focused and slightly intimidated by the task ahead, but I was determined to rise to the whole challenging scenario.

Many mistakes can be attributed to a 'system' failure rather than to any one person or problem. Such system failures occur when individual actions or problems 'slip through the net' for one reason or another, and one small incident or lapse can pave the way for the next, which compounds the error and increases the likelihood of it culminating in an episode of harm affecting the patient. This scenario is compared to holes in a block of Swiss cheese. When the holes line up, a process can progress through the holes in the block of cheese from beginning to end, without being caught by any of the safety features in the system.

That day the holes in the cheese began lining up early on.

I was unsure what constituted a heavy pre-med. Although only 12 years old, John was large and overweight. Despite this, he looked cute having a dark floppy fringe and a big smile: he looked happy and content. I erred on the side of caution and prescribed a dose of the only sedative I knew for use in children.

It was not until later that it was clearly, a thoroughly inadequate dose. The ward telephoned down to theatre mid morning to notify us that John was very distressed and threatening to leave the hospital. The pre-med did not seem to be working and Mum was angry: she had been assured this would not happen again.

John and his mother were brought down to theatre reception shortly afterwards and I went round to apologise face to face for the inadequate sedation and subsequent distress. In an attempt to salvage the situation I ventured to reception armed with a cannula to insert into his hand and a syringe containing intravenous sedative agent, ready to give. John was protesting, loudly refusing to come to the anaesthetic room. I approached keeping my cannula hidden. I reassured John with a small lie, saying he would not have to go to the anaesthetic room, *if* he would allow me just one attempt at cannulation on the back of his chubby hand. Unexpectedly, he agreed to this. He would need it inserted before general anaesthesia anyway, so doing it in advance of the anaesthetic room merely expedited proceedings. I was pleased to see the ward nurses had applied the magic cream to numb the back of his hands, despite me not remembering to prescribe it.

I knew I would not get a second chance to put the needle into his hand but lady luck fleetingly appeared at my side and the cannula slid perfectly into the vein. I quickly followed it up with a substantial dose of the sedative I had brought with me ready prepared.

Anxious not to make the same mistake twice, this time I gave a larger than average dose of the drug, a fast acting sedative which also causes memory loss for events occurring subsequently.

It did what it said on the tin and John became unable to protest further. Grabbing the opportunity we quickly wheeled him round to the anaesthetic room on the trolley. I was aware he was heavily sedated and unmonitored but he was breathing well and was safe. My focus was on maintaining my advantage and getting the anaesthetic into him as quickly as possible and definitely before he had a chance to rouse again. Still quiescent as we entered the anaesthetic room, I clamped the mask to his face and turned on the gas. Only the slightest concentration of gas was required to render him fully anaesthetised.

With the patient and the frantic situation now under control, there was a collective sigh of relief. He could no longer abscond and would now definitely have his problematic toenail removed. Silently, I congratulated myself on this achievement, noting that Mum too, looked pleased. She thanked us as she left the anaesthetic room leaving the care of her son up to us.

By now we were running behind schedule so we continued to rush, whisking the patient into theatre where the surgeon was already getting scrubbed up. John had kept one bed sock on and the exposed toe was efficiently painted with iodine by the scrub nurse and draped to maintain a sterile field.

Seconds later the surgeon appeared at the table and without delay he removed the toenail in one swift move. Before I had even written any notes, it was over and he was bandaging the toe up. I switched off the gas to allow the patient to wake up gradually, knowing it would take some time after the recent, generous dose of pre-operative sedation.

An auxiliary nurse was gathering up the patient's belongings. She found the second sock under the trolley and to pair it up with it's partner, whipped the other sock off the foot on the non-operated side.

It was then we saw it. The red swollen infected great toenail on the opposite foot, previously kept hidden and protected under a sock.

The patient was almost awake but I deepened the anaesthesia easily so he remained asleep while we had a heated discussion about how this had happened and who was to blame.

The surgeon was a man of few words and was in no mood for reflection. With the job not yet done he proceeded to repeat the same process on the opposite side and remove the correct toenail. I thought this was the sensible thing to do: that toenail was the cause of the original problem after all, it was the first toenail, the normal one, that had been removed in error.

The patient arrived in recovery with two matching bandaged big toes.

Without any discussion between us, the surgeon immediately summoned Mum and explained that the other toenail, (the one removed in error) had also looked to be developing the same problem so he had decided to do the procedure on both sides at the same time, particularly given the previous pre-operative difficulties. I listened, feeling well out of my depth and wishing we had rehearsed our speech in advance. I did not know my lines, or even if I had a speaking part! Should I speak up and tell the truth or remain complicit with silence? I remained unsure whether to speak or not and also what I would say? I didn't want to contradict the surgeon nor show him to be lying. I decided it was best to keep quiet.

Mum was profuse in her thanks to the surgeon and extremely grateful that neither she nor her son would have to go through this same procedure in the future.

At that time I thought the surgeon was heroic and inventive. By cleverly justifying his actions he had gotten away with it. As the years passed since then, I have become less comfortable with his dishonest explanation and failure to admit responsibility for the error. Removal of the normal toenail was not necessary and technically would constitute an assault on the patient in the view taken by the courts. However, the fabricated explanation given to his mother sounded reasonable and she happily accepted it. The outcome could easily have been far more messy and acrimonious for all concerned.

A difficult patient had caused us all to deviate from our normal protocols and checking procedures as our priority was to get on with the operation. No one had checked which side was to be operated on and no one had removed the remaining sock. The outcome is all too easy to predict now, with the benefit of hindsight.

My overwhelming feeling was one of relief. Relief that it wasn't me who had done anything wrong. Relief that I was not to blame. But theatre is a team sport and I had played a part; my well-meaning top up of sedation in reception had set the wheels in motion for mistakes to happen as we collectively focussed on controlling the situation and rushing the patient to theatre.

The following 20 years would see a proliferation of peri-operative checklists and procedures put in place to stop these very occurrences. I often wonder how the same scenario would pan out in today's systems. I suspect a junior anaesthetist would not have taken the matter into her own hands and would have referred the patient to a consultant to deal with. I learnt a lot from this experience and I believe I made the correct decision, acting in the best interests of the patient at all times.

10. No Bleepin' Privacy

Having a bleep is a great accolade and is loved by all junior doctors. How important we feel when it goes off! Somebody wants us, no, somebody *needs* us, no-one else will do. Of course, we let it bleep as many times as possible before reading the number to call. We then pretend it's an annoying intrusion. 'What do they want *now?*' We sigh. It is hard being so busy and important enough that everyone wants you. We feel quite indispensable.

All too soon though, reality bites and the bleep displays it's true colours. It becomes a nuisance. It interrupts. Its piercing tone reminds you that you are at the beck and call of others who deem their need is more important than anything else you may be doing. Perhaps that's why it is called a bleep! The bleep can insist you make contact with any number of others at all times of day and night, confirming that there is no such thing as privacy in hospitals.

This is bad enough for the patients who have no choice about being in hospital and it is not much better for us doctors who work there. Although we are not unwell, wearing a flimsy gown or suffering acute pain, we are subject to on call rooms that don't lock, grill fronted lockers where contents lie visible in the changing rooms and at least one bleep to ensure a variety of people know exactly where you are and perhaps what you are doing at any given moment.

When on call it is usual to have a 'bedroom' on intensive care. It means you are in close proximity to the patients should you be needed in an emergency. It also means you are easily available to the nurses.

I use the word 'bedroom' in the loosest possible sense: there would be a bed and there would be sheets on it (although these may or may not have been changed from the previous night's occupant). There would be curtains but not always a window as previously mentioned. There would be a telephone and if you were really lucky it would reach from the socket to the bedside, meaning you did not have to get out of bed to answer your bleep. This is a particular nuisance when the call is only for advice and does not necessitate you getting out of bed. The same applied to the lamp. Sometimes it too would be close enough to the bed so it could be switched on (to look at the numbers on your bleep), without getting out of bed. Such little things made a huge difference to the annoyance factor of being on call.

In the past I'm sure doctors were brought extra blankets from matron on night shift and tea and toast from the nurses at 6am (universal hospital toast time, always wonderful, white bread dripping with butter) but those days passed very early in my career. Now, rather than inconvenience the nurses by having them bleep you, if they want your services, they can instead just phone you or they can knock on your bedroom door directly. No need to worry about being asleep and not hearing the knock: if you don't answer immediately they will promptly open the door and give you a verbal nudge. Sometimes the door will even have a square glass panel in it so they can peer through it without alerting you to their presence. (Until they have confirmed you are really asleep before they wake you up!). That's how it feels anyway.

Sometimes I wondered if there was a spy cam by the wash hand basin. Each time I began to brush my teeth in anticipation of going to bed, my bleep would go off, bleeping, flashing, vibrating, laughing?

Needless to say such bedrooms do not feel like homely secure retreats. In the morning, following a 24 hour period at the beck and call of nurses, patients, casualty doctors, and any other doctor who had a patient that required more than a quick glance, it was a relief to go home to my own bed safe in the knowledge than no-one would or could wake me up before *I* decided it was time to wake up. It brought a feeling of a great freedom and an almost physical lightness upon leaving the hospital. I loved the anticipation of going home for a hot shower and a bowl of rice crispies while my electric blanket warmed the bed.

Being tied to the job on a short leash was okay for much of the time and it wasn't always as bad as it sounds. At other times though, the lack of privacy and the demands of others for attention was soul destroying.

On one intensive care unit, the staff toilet was housed within a wooden pillar structure close to the entrance of the unit. The walls were paper thin and it was only used by staff on breaks who had no time to walk the 500 yards along the corridor to the facilities in the changing room. You could hear everything through these walls which I found fairly inhibitory to the smooth emptying of one's bladder. I avoided using this toilet whenever possible but this day, when I realised the sound travelled equally in both directions, I had no choice.I had been busy all day not stopping for a drink or a loo break. It is common to reach the end of a day at work and realise that you have not passed urine all day and actually really need to go! As was now the case.

As I entered and locked the toilet door, I heard a patient's relatives at the nurses desk asking if they could speak with the doctor on duty. That was me. I could sense the nurse scanning the unit before saying 'she was here a moment ago, I'm not sure where she has gone, but she won't be far away'.

As she shouted to a colleague regarding my whereabouts I stood still. I really needed to go. Should I go and speak to the relatives and come back later? Talking with relatives is never a quick job, nor can it be rushed. I might not last. Should I go quickly, aware that they may hear me emptying my bladder from the short distance between us? Why was I embarrassed by this thought? I am a doctor for heaven's sake and it is a normal bodily function! I had to go, so go I did.

Just as I sat down and began to relax, my pager went off.

The insistent beep beep, rigorous vibration and flashing red light ensured that it would always alert you even if asleep, in a noisy environment, blind or deaf.

Transiently I felt relieved; the sound of my bleeper would drown out the sounds of toileting. My relief quickly evaporated however, when I heard the same nurse tell the relatives 'Oh, I can hear her pager go off, she's just in the toilet. Shouldn't be too long'.

No matter how comfortable you are about bodily functions, it still does not feel right to have relatives of critically unwell patients, waiting for you to emerge from the loo. Surely they will be unable to help but think about what you were doing in there?

I washed my hands thoroughly. Should I leave them slightly wet to reassure them I had washed them? Or would this make them suspicious they were wet from contamination and had not been washed? Suddenly all these tiny issues appeared from nowhere and seemed incredibly important. The line between me being the doctor on duty and me just being plain old me, going to the toilet like everyone else was faint. The two sides did not blend comfortably.

The solution I chose was to be professional and deal with them in my normal manner. I introduced myself, moved to a quiet room and asked how I could help, without reference to the delay, the noises coming from the toilet or their invasion of my personal space and time.

The truth is when on call you have no personal time to call your own. You are literally 'on call' for the whole period. Unlike nurses who get regular breaks (but are not paid during those 15 minute periods), doctors get no such protected breaks when on duty. This works both ways of course and when life is busy we are rushed off our feet with barely enough time to eat, drink and void. The flip side is that when it is quiet, we can use the time as we choose. We make the most of it too, well aware that the longer it lasts, the more likely it is to be brought to an abrupt end by anyone of a variety of people demanding your time and attention.

For patients the lack of privacy is even more of an issue. I am never surprised by the prevalence of constipation amongst inpatients using a bed pan behind screens in a six bedded bay, being asked if they are finished every two minutes. I wonder why we pull the curtains around the bed space before a patient consultation? Are we implying that if we can't be seen, we won't be heard? My voice carries clearly despite the curtains and my direct questions, as well as the patients answers are heard by the other five patients who pretend to be engrossed in their reading. Such embarrassing lack of privacy is far from ideal and can be detrimental to the doctor patient relationship.

Some patients take extreme measures to ensure privacy and anonymity. I was called to see a patient who needed to come to theatre as soon as possible. As I carried out my pre-operative assessment I marvelled at the lack of luck this man had. Dr Peters was a GP and worked in a neighbouring area. He had not wished to present to his local hospital due to fear of being known and recognised by staff and patients alike, so he had driven several miles to come to the hospital where I was working.

Earlier in the evening there had been an accident. Dr Peters had been relaxing at home when he tripped and fell into his vegetable rack. He had fallen awkwardly, knocking over the rack, sending vegetables flying in all directions. He landed on a cucumber which plunged into his back passage and had become firmly impacted in his rectum. (He had removed his trousers and underwear earlier because he spilt coffee on them. He was en route to put them into the washing machine when he slipped. Just in case you were wondering.)

When the casualty doctor examined him, the end of the cucumber was not visible nor palpable and could not be simply removed. He was referred to the surgeons.

Next came a telephone call from the police. Had Dr Peters been brought in?

Dr Peters' wife had arrived home and been alarmed to find the house empty. As time passed and it grew dark she became increasingly worried. His mobile phone was switched off and he was not with any of his usual friends. The car was gone from the drive and she feared the worst. She reported this to the police and a check around local hospitals had begun.

Dr Peters reassured them he was indeed here and everything was fine. No, his wife need not attend; it was far too late and his stomach cramps were settling. He was sure he would be discharged shortly.

There was a significant wait for the surgeon to come and review Dr Peters and it was after 11pm when he arrived. After another examination and failed attempt to reach the cucumber, he decided to take Dr Peters to theatre to remove the cucumber from the bowel. If left, there was a risk of bowel perforation and catastrophic damage. The intention of a quick trip to hospital to get the offending object pulled out with a long pair of graspers had not worked out as planned by Dr Peters.

In theatre, anaesthesia was induced without problem and the first plan was to use a telescope to remove the object. With the patient's legs held up and apart in the stirrups, the black telescope snaked into his rectum and upwards to the colon. Unfortunately, the cucumber had migrated further in and was positioned awkwardly, the ends neither free nor visible. There was nothing for forceps to grab hold of. The next step was to convert to an open operation. Inside the abdomen the bowel could be incised to remove the cucumber safely.

It is so true that once you have told one lie, you must keep telling lies to make the story remain plausible. I wondered what Mrs Peters was going to be told now? With his legs now down flat on the operating table, Dr Peters' abdomen was cleaned and prepped for surgery while the surgeons scrubbed up at the sinks.

Inside the abdomen, the affected piece of bowel looked distended and the smell was not pleasant. The wall of the bowel had been pierced by one end of the cucumber allowing bowel contents to leak into the abdomen. This is never a good thing. After removal of the cucumber and copious washing out of the abdominal cavity, the next decision brought Dr Peters even more bad luck.

Due to the leakage and contamination from the punctured bowel, it was not safe to join up the two ends of the bowel again. Instead, a temporising measure was performed that brought out to the surface of the abdomen not one, but two stomas. Complete with plastic collection bags attached. This would allow time for infection to clear and makes repair of the bowel at a later date more likely to succeed. Things could not have turned out any worse for Dr Peters. Or perhaps they could.

By now it was the middle of the night and the next telephone call from the police confirmed that Mrs Peters was on her way to the hospital, concerned about what had happened to her husband. I hoped her concern remained when she heard of the evening's events and lasted through to his next operation to join the bowel back up, at some point in the future.

When Dr Peters awoke, the lack of privacy and anonymity would be the least of his worries.

The lack of privacy becomes more serious when it impacts upon patient confidentiality. This is magnified in rural areas where patients are treated in their local hospital and they know, or know of, many of the staff. The reverse is also true, with many staff and patients of comparable ages having grown up together or attending the same school.

I saw Mrs B in a typical six bedded bay. She was small and timid, fidgeting with the edge of her cardigan; her posture was hunched over and she kept her eyes down, as if trying to disappear within herself. She was slightly odd and reticent when it came to divulging her medical history and I had a feeling she was keeping something back. A few probing questions yielded no positive findings and after deciding she was fit for her proposed operation and general anaesthetic I tried a final 'Is there anything else you think I should know?' but with no response I mentally shrugged and left the ward.

When she arrived in theatre reception the next day, she requested to speak with me again. I went out to the trolley bay and drew the curtains around to 'exclude' the two other male patients who had arrived for their operations too. Again Mrs B seemed strange, embarrassed and uneasy. She asked me if she was going to be alright. Thinking she was merely anxious, I reassured her swiftly and brought her around to my anaesthetic room without further ado. After siting the cannula in her hand, I was about to begin giving the anaesthetic drugs when she stopped me in my tracks and asked 'Can I speak to you alone first?' I looked at my anaesthetic nurse and the auxiliary present. Both stepped outside and Mrs B began.

'I'm being investigated for a rare inherited disorder at the genetics clinic in the city. I don't want my family to know or to find out why I'm here. So far I've seen a nurse who lives on my street and my niece was here visiting her friend. I wanted to tell you in private. I don't know if it's important for my anaesthetic.'

In a hospital where the paths of staff and patients can cross in various different roles it is understandably difficult for patients to be assured of privacy and confidentiality. It is a fact we are aware of and take seriously to prevent important information being withheld by the patient to the detriment of their care.

11. Lies, Lies and More Lies

Patients tell lies to their doctors all the time and it is no different with anaesthetists. Some lies told by patients are not that important: do they smoke? How much do they drink? When asking these questions we almost always know the ball park the true answer falls within.

Sometimes though, lies can cause catastrophic consequences, (as opposed to mere embarrassment as suffered by Dr Peters and the cucumber.) Patients lie about what they have had to eat and drink preceding surgery, or more accurately what they haven't had to eat and drink. Knowing they were supposed to fast for a period prior to the operation, they are wise enough to know their operation will be postponed or cancelled if they have not fasted appropriately.

Why do they lie?

I can testify from personal experience, that fasting with no food or drink is a hard and unpleasant experience and we do not demand this of patients for fun. Nor is it some form of punitive exercise. The reason there are strict fasting guidelines is for patient safety. Neither party wants the situation where one of them is picking lumps of toast, curry or anything else, from the other's lungs. If the stomach is not devoid of food and liquid when anaesthesia is induced, there is a good chance the contents will regurgitate back up the gullet, seep into the windpipe and subsequently burn the lungs with gastric acid. Under anaesthesia, this regurgitation of stomach contents will not induce the normal responses of coughing, choking or vomiting. It will go where gravity takes it. Anything in the lungs which is not supposed to be there induces inflammatory and infective processes to develop and prevents normal lung function. Again, this is never a good thing.

As well as foods, patients often deny any substance abuse. I understand many of their reasons for this: their parents are present, I might cancel their operation (I will), I might tell the police (I won't), they want to believe their muscles are due entirely to gym work, or taking the substance is now such a normal part of their life they don't regard it as a problem. They may not think to mention it or choose not to mention it as they don't see how it matters. Well, it does matter, a lot.

Illegal substances can have severe and unpredictable effects on the heart and circulation. It is nice to be forewarned of these and to look at the heart rhythm beforehand, deciding if the benefit of the proposed surgery merits the risk that will be taken.

Cynically perhaps, I have a low level of suspicion for drug use and ask about it routinely, in a casual manner: it doesn't bother me whether they do or don't take illegal substances but I like to know what I'm dealing with when I take responsibility for their life and try very hard to get all the relevant information.

When faced with a body builder I ask about any supplements they take. What they are called and where they have come from. Many dangerous cocktails can be bought over the internet, marketed as 'supplements' when in fact they contain potent stimulants. This was partly discovered as the number of reports of fit, young body builders suffering bizarre cardiac rhythms during induction of anaesthesia increased. Several such individuals have died as a direct result of this, having attended for minor elective surgery. This is a tragedy made worse by knowing their deaths were due to their non-disclosure of medications they were taking and were ultimately preventable.

My gut feeling was on red alert when I first met Mark. All the clues were present and although it would be politically incorrect to say so, his extensive tattoos, disgusting dentition and stab wound courtesy of 'his mate' for 'doin' nuhin' increased my suspicion. His personality was not my favourite either. Wearing tracksuit bottoms with a naked torso he lay back against his pillows, hands clasped behind his head, hirsute arm pits on full display. His default facial expression was a smirk and he exuded contempt.

'Mark Henderson?' I confirmed as I approached his bed holding the notes.

'Aawwwwrrrright pal,' came the reply. I ignored this inappropriate over-familiarity and shuddered to think of being his 'pal'. It was not worth insisting to be addressed as Doctor, sometimes you have to choose your battles. I repeated my question.

'Depends who's askin' an' all doan it?' I ignored this too and carried on, deciding to keep the questions brief and direct, restricting myself to asking only the bare essentials and getting the unpleasant consultation over with as quickly as possible.

When I'm suspicious of the patient being an illicit drug user, my conversation follows a well used script This consultation was textbook and I smiled inwardly at my small victory when the predictable outcome resulted.

'Do you take any medicines?'

'No.'

'Are you allergic to anything?'

'No.'

'You don't take any medicines or drugs?' I sound surprised.

'No.'

'No drugs at all? Nothing prescribed by your doctor?'

'No.'

'Anything *not* prescribed by your doctor?'

'No.'

'Not even weed or anything?' I now sound incredulous, as if I *know* that everyone smokes some weed but I'm so cool I wholly endorse it. (I expect I am years behind with the terminology; do people still call it weed?)

'Good,' I reassure him. 'The reason I ask is that some drugs mean you need more of the anaesthetic to keep you fully asleep.'

This is not untrue. Many illicit drugs induce enzymes in the body making it much more efficient at metabolising drugs used during anaesthesia, thus making them effective for a much shorter period of time.

Without hesitation I move on and ask the rest of my questions. At the end of the consultation, when some thinking time has elapsed and questions are invited, there is commonly a small quiet voice that asks 'What you were saying earlier...about the drugs...does smoking weed matter?'

'No, not really but thanks for mentioning it. Anything else at all that you take, even occasionally?' and then the truth, the whole extent of the truth comes pouring out, because we're pals now, right?

12. The Motivated Patient

There has been an explosion in the use of day surgery and shorter stay 24 hour surgery in recent years. The driver for this has been bed closures on the ward (to keep costs down) and has been facilitated by improved surgical techniques and shorter acting anaesthetic agents, both of which promote faster recovery. Despite costing more than traditional methods and equipment, this way is cheaper than an overnight in hospital (or the money comes from a different budget so any increased cost will not be visible for this exercise).

A lot of effort is put into achieving a post operative patient who is in a fit state to go home the same day or early the day after surgery. The patient is seen at clinic beforehand and optimally prepared to allow admission on the same day they have their surgery. Patients carry out the some of the required preparation at home by shaving relevant areas, changing their diet as instructed or consuming some powerful bowel emptying powder.

The surgery is efficient and slick, achieved by having a senior surgeon perform the operation, carefully selecting the patients and doing only operations predicted to be straight forward. The pain relief is generous and varied to block pain pathways from many different angles. No expense is spared with the anti-sickness medication. Fluid balance is maintained, temperature is corrected, progress in the recovery room is actively managed. Protocols and guidelines proliferate to ensure the current thinking in best practice is followed.

Despite all this effort, sometimes it happens that a patient may not be fit to be discharged home the same day and needs to be admitted to a hospital bed for on-going care. It is almost impossible to predict the patients who will require this; there are so many variables. Conversely, the opposite group, the patients who are always up, fit and ready to leave, are easy to identify.

These are the motivated patients, identified by having at least one of the following characteristics. Firstly, they work either on a part time basis or are self employed. Either way they do not get any sick pay and being able to work is very important to them. Secondly, they are smokers. These patients are always up and about, grinning and bearing it, eager to go home. This is also borne out over in the maternity ward where recovery after Caesarean section is much faster in smokers. Money and addiction are the two biggest motivators in life and in medicine it is no different.

While it would be ironical if cigarettes were the key to shortening patient stay in hospital, this merely illustrates the profound effect that a patient's motivation has on their outcome. Those who want to or need to get out of bed do so much more quickly than those who have no such incentive

The other instance where patient motivation is relevant is regarding needles. Nobody likes needles. Fact. But some mind them less than others and some mind them even less when they are to ink a tattoo. When it comes to the dentist, or the 'needle' in the back of the hand (which is actually a plastic tube) some mind it so much they define themselves as needle phobic. There are a few true needle phobics around and these people have my sympathy (and they do not have tattoos or piercings) but just as needles are necessary for tattoos, so too are they needed for many medical procedures. Anaesthesia is a non starter if there is no 'needle in the vein'. There is no choice for those who wish to proceed with their operation: eggs and omelettes spring to mind. Some patients insist they are needle phobic and request to breathe the gas to go to sleep, a technique usually reserved for children. This may or may not be agreed to by the anaesthetist because this technique is not as simple in an adult as it is in a child. The risks of going to sleep this way are certainly different and most likely increased.

Motivated patients do not mind needles and those in severe pain barely notice them. A labouring woman requesting an epidural for pain relief barely notices the large cannula being inserted into her hand first. In fact, the response to inserting this cannula is now my way to diagnose true labour, before I site the epidural. Those presenting for purely aesthetic surgery rarely mention any needle phobias and those presenting covered in tattoos from head to toe are not given much sympathy whatever they say, I'm afraid.

13. A Good Teacher

During training we learn through mentorship and professional example. Although the curriculum consists of many technical skills and procedures to be mastered, there remains a healthy degree of apprenticeship where we learn the *conduct* of anaesthesia; bringing together all the skills, including non technical skills so that the operating list runs smoothly. We learn professional behaviour, attitudes and organisational skills by following the examples set by our consultant trainers. Much of this comes from being doubled up on theatre lists with the wise old owls of the department. Those who have seen it all, can handle anything, and never appear fazed. For them, the technicalities of the job are practically automatic, and certainly stress free, so they like to amuse themselves in theatre, holding court particularly to new members of staff or visitors who have not heard their jokes before.

With each individual's practice that you observe during the training years, you tend to adopt the good bits and learn how to avoid the bad bits, or leave them by the wayside. I fondly remember the director of the intensive care unit I first worked on. We worked to his rules and I will always remember them.

'If the kidneys fail, we can filter the patient, if the lungs fail, he dies'. This served to focus our prescribing of judicious fluids and not 'drowning the lungs'. Another mantra, which stands true to this day was 'No diagnosis, no chance'. Intensive care can prop up every failing organ system in the body (except the brain) but without an accurate diagnosis and specific, direct treatment, the patient will not get better.

To solve diagnostic dilemmas he told us we could 'Explain the mystery by revisiting the history'. Reminding us to 'ask the correct questions and listen very carefully to the story of the illness'. (More than nine out of ten diagnoses are made upon the history alone. Subsequent examination and hi-tech investigations only serve to confirm these pointers and our initial suspicions.) We see this in action in intensive care: the patient rarely gets better when we treat the symptoms alone, when we don't know the cause of the problems we are treating. 'Stable' on intensive care is not good. It means the patient is deteriorating. 'We are providing intensive, expensive, round the clock treatment, the patient ought to be improving' he would emphasise, as if it was our fault the patient was no better. He had high standards and commanded respect throughout the hospital, throughout the country in fact and I definitely received a thorough grounding and insight into an awe-inspiring side of hospital medicine from him.

To this day, I can hear the wise words Dr Roberts shared with me as a novice anaesthetist in theatre too. As I learnt to insert devices to prop open the airway he would demand 'Precision technique, attention to detail and a perfect fit' stating these would prevent problems developing with a laryngeal mask airway, sitting over the vocal cords. 'Never settle for anything less' he warned. It is as memorable as it is true. Sloppy technique *does* cause problems, problems that we often *do* get away with, but not always. I think of him with a smile each time I rush a procedure and decide it's 'probably okay' and 'will do for now', hoping his motto will not come back to haunt me.

The community dental list is always a challenge in many respects. It consists of children, with neglected, carious teeth for extraction. It was sad to see such advanced decay in pre-school age children, usually from the lower socio-economic classes, commonly with fizzy drinks in baby feeding bottles, bathing their teeth in sugar and acid, and keep them quiet I suspect.

My first teacher on this list was humorous in a way that others found disconcerting. Dead pan, he would look at the child on the dental list and say 'Oh, so you've been drinking fizzy juice? That could mix with the anaesthetic gases and make you explode!' his eyes wide and voice serious, 'we'll need to post pone your operation until it empties from your tummy because we don't want an explosion to make a mess in the theatre.'

The parents were not exempt from his humour.

'You're the best mum we've had all morning' he would say to the tearful parent as her young child was rendered floppy and unresponsive from the syringe of magic milk medicine. It was funny when said to the parent of the first child, and even funnier when he repeated to the dad accompanying the second child.

What did I learn from him? I'm not sure exactly but it was an insight into the fun that can be had, though wrong on so many levels, when you have the privilege of being a doctor.

Anaesthesia is often cited as an excellent specialty for women. What people really mean when they say this is that it is good specialty if you want to work less than full time (part time to you and me). In a lot of ways this is true, the work is sessional and the duty of care finite. When we go home at the end of each day our on call team will deal with problems arising or a need to return to theatre for all patients.

I remember fondly one consultant trainer I had who was explaining to the awestruck, female, medical student in the anaesthetic room with us that day that anaesthesia was a good specialty for women. He confirmed this with a serious nod saying women often felt at home in the anaesthetic room. Knowing him well, I awaited the punch line.

'Look around you,' he continued 'doesn't it make you feel relaxed? Doesn't it give you a sense of security and familiarity?' he asked dead pan. Looking puzzled the medical student was unsure how to respond. She was embarrassed and looked at me for help, but I didn't know where this was going either. She elected to remain silent.

'Of course you do! Look! There are worktops! Well stocked cupboards! A sink! Even a little fridge. We are all wearing rubber gloves, and even the suction! Look! It works just like a little hoover...'

While setting women's equality in the workplace back several decades and not being in anyway politically correct, this was incredibly funny. This is an accurate description of the anaesthetic room and joking aside, the whole concept is not too far from the truth. You see, anaesthesia *is* a bit like housework. When it is done well, no-one notices it. Everyone is happy. The surgeon is happy to be able to get on with his operation, the recovery staff are happy that the patient is pain free, and the ward staff are happy when a big drip is left in place and the on-going plan for fluids and pain relief is prescribed. Most important of all, the patients are happy. They are happy because they went to sleep, stayed asleep, and woke up at the end. If you're a real anaesthetic domestic goddess they won't feel sick or complain of pain either. Result.

In contrast, when no anaesthetist turns up all hell breaks loose. Crisis management is deployed as unanswered bleeps lead to phone calls to department secretaries, who shuffle other anaesthetists around and redeploy someone to fill the gap, and the lists start late, if at all. Yes, people would notice if it wasn't done at all.

However, like housework, it is when anaesthesia is done badly that everything starts to unravel. The conduct of anaesthesia is not a tangible entity. The differences between a slick and a not so slick anaesthetic are subtle. Tiny details may not be individually apparent but add up to become significant. If not timed to perfection the patient may move or cough. This annoys the surgeons no end so can be worthwhile doing once in a while, (just don't try it during eye surgery)! To remedy the situation may require additional drugs which may then delay the eventual process of awakening. While fast is not always better, surgeons love a fast anaesthetist because time is precious in theatre and they hate hanging around waiting for us. However, we are a necessary evil if they want to perform surgery.

Sub-optimal pain relief means the patient is remanded in the recovery room being pumped full of morphine, quickly followed by anti-sickness drugs, sick bowls and cold soaked paper towels on their foreheads. (No, no idea why.) If you've really messed it up in the day surgery unit, the patient may need admitted overnight, which defeats the objective of day surgery. Everything gets a bit messy and then people start to notice. They phone you, they want you to attend, they want you to be aware, they just want to let you know. This all takes time, causes delay, causes over-running lists. This annoys the theatre sister, who pesters the surgeon, who blames the anaesthetist. The chaos evolves.

Of course patients don't have anaesthetics for the sake of it. They don't present to hospital for an anaesthetic. They present wanting or needing an operation. Let us not forget our raison d'etre. But anaesthetising a surgical list is more than putting the patients to sleep and waking them up again. It is managing the list to run efficiently, planning, organising, facilitating the smooth running of the day's proceedings, working towards the common goal. This pivotal role can easily go unnoticed, particularly when done well. Some theatres just seem to work well though while others are beset by delays, moans and problems.

I consider it a great success to fly below the radar, quietly and effectively getting on with it. If no-one notices me or what I have done, it means things have been smooth and the patient stable. I do not expect a round of applause if I have done a good job, which is just as well really!. While the surgeons receive letters and gifts from grateful patients with new hips and knees, I am happy to be long forgotten by patients and pleased to remain anonymous.

Another consultant liked to amuse his audience in the anaesthetic room, usually at the patient's expense though not in any malicious way. It is usual practice to give patients pure oxygen to breathe before they go to sleep. This is delivered through a mask which we hold over their mouth and nose and instruct them to take deep breaths.

'Deep breaths, nice deep breaths, pretend this is your first cigarette of the morning and you want to get as much as you can into your lungs' he would say, laughing.

Other times it would be 'Big breaths, nice big breaths for me, that's it' or to take it a step further 'Big breasts now, nice big breasts for me, that's good, big breasts...' Cue school boy snickering from all males in the room, every time.

Other teachers are memorable for altogether different reasons. As an assertive woman in medicine it is easy to become labelled as 'stroppy' or 'feisty' and some are more deserving of this descriptor than others. Dr Deborah was one such consultant.

She was a petite Irish woman, quite new to our department but an established consultant with many years experience. She was well respected but we as trainees found her a bit scary. She *was* a bit abrupt. She took no prisoners and was not to be messed with.There was no joking or innuendo in her anaesthetic room.

One afternoon I was doubled up with her in theatre so we met at lunchtime to discuss the patients. Her bleep went off displaying the number for the ward we had just left and as she answered it I realised it was the surgical trainee on the other end of the line. Paul was a friend of mine. He was loud and funny and I liked him a lot. We had worked together in casualty and now he was pursuing a surgical career. He confided in me that since starting surgery his favourite part of the operation was the very end. I assumed this was because he got to practice stitching up the wounds but no, he explained, it was because he'd noticed that prior to waking the patients up, the anaesthetists always lean forwards to clear the back of the patients' throat with the suction. This meant he could see right down the front of their tops. I realised then why so many had tape across the baggy V neck theatre tops and made a note to be careful of this in future.

This day, I heard him begin the conversation:

'Hi, about Jeannie who you're gassing first this afternoon...'

'No. I'm not.' came the retort. I cringed for him as he was cut short.

'Err, yes, you are!? You're Dr Deborah aren't you? Your name's on the list.'

Her face showed an icy calm.

'I am aware of who I am and what the afternoon rota shows but I am not *gassing* anyone this afternoon' she articulated. 'If you want to discuss the anaesthesia for one of your patients I suggest you come down here, introduce yourself, and speak to me with a little respect.' The phone slammed down and I felt sorry for Paul being on the receiving end of such a sharp tongue while knowing that it would be water off a duck's back to him; I could imagine him mumbling 'Must be her time of the month,' or something similar in his off hand manner.

It is easy to make others feel small and inferior in medicine and many do this to make themselves sound big and important. A definite hierarchy is present and you can usually find someone on the rungs below you. The way you treat them is often a sign of your own confidence or lack thereof. Some doctors act the way their seniors acted towards them in 'the good old days' and others remember how awful it was to be intimidated in this manner and are much more civil and understanding. For the rest, it really depends which side of bed they got out of that morning.

14. Shoes

As a final year medical student in obstetrics, one of the requirements was that we had to deliver (well, help deliver) at least 10 babies. This was quite a challenge given the short time we were to spend there, the unpredictability of the delivery time and the propensity of mammals to deliver their young at unsociable hours, in the safety of darkness. We needed our logbooks signed off by the midwife present at the birth. This too was a challenge on many levels.

The relationship between midwifery staff and medical staff is fragile at best. Predominantly, the hostility of midwives is directed towards the obstetricians, those doctors who try to ruin natural childbirth with medical intervention (but also those whom they call to take responsibility for anything not going quite as well as expected), but in truth, they can make life difficult for anyone falling under the umbrella of 'medical staff'. Including medical students. In fact, we were easy fodder: way out of our comfort zone, right into theirs. We needed to be there and while they tolerated our presence, they made it clear we were in their way.

Choosing a patient in labour whose baby you may be allowed to help deliver was a lucky dip. You wanted the women who would have fast, normal labours and would deliver a healthy baby promptly, preferably before dinner time. Ideally, she would be under the care of a tick box happy midwife. The chances of this happening are akin to hoping for a sunny day in the UK, when you are not working and have a barbecue planned. Slim to none. Instead we would frequently find ourselves allocated to a woman having labour induced, augmented with uterine stimulants, continuous fetal monitoring in place, a prolonged second stage of pushing but no progress, and after 10 hours of small talk with the couple, as you hung on awaiting the grand finale, it would culminate in a trip to theatre for a Caesarean section, depriving you of notching up a delivery on your card. How inconsiderate. A whole day wasted. Even when you thought you had chosen well, the nature of childbirth is fickle and all can change in an instant.

I must not fail to mention that on labour ward the attire is the same blue scrubs as worn in the operating theatre. It too has changing room obstacles as mentioned earlier but, by the fifth and final year of university we were much better at getting changed and getting into the workplace, and could still recognise people 'without their clothes on'. Oh how we laughed at that.

The problem of footwear remained. As visiting students we were not given our own theatre shoes (this would be a waste of resources) so we had to make do with those lying around in the changing room and hope that they were truly spare and sore feet was the only thing we caught from them.

One day I found a matching pair, the name of the owner written on both heels. I was now theatre-shoe-wise, bolder than at my first disastrous venture into theatre and reckoned it was safe to assume their owner was not at work, or she would have been wearing her shoes by now. I decided they were to be mine for the day.

Of course it was a longer rather than a shorter day. Tempting though it was to duck out of the labouring couples' room and give them some privacy, there remained the fear that the midwife would not sign your card unless you had been involved in the entire experience. It is called 'labour' for very good reasons for both the mother and the medical student! After a whole day of waiting, tedium filled with breathing exercises and sojourns from the bed to the bouncy ball, it finally seemed as if delivery of a baby was imminent so I decided to hang on into the evening and catch the delivery.

Time continued to pass and progress slowed as it approached the finale. It grew dark outside and it was now too late to consider dinner. Babies are considerate creatures and never arrive during the change of shift or dare to interrupt the sacrosanct 'handover report'. There is a general hiatus in all activity as the night staff arrive but have yet to formally take over.

I became aware that my midwife was looking at her watch and mumbling to herself around the same time as the altercation outside the door grew louder.

It seemed one of the night staff could not find her shoes in the changing room and it was suspected someone had 'borrowed' them. I quickly realised it was going to be me and by now knew the drill. I could not escape to the changing rooms or I might miss the delivery so I waited for my dressing down. It did not disappoint. Full of 'Who did I think I was?' and 'How dare I'. I stood my ground and waited for the storm to pass noting how much thicker my skin had become in the last two years. I could ride it out; see this baby delivered, get my card signed and get the hell out of there. I would soon forget all about another faceless midwife screaming at a member of medical staff.

I was in my final year and such petty conflicts no longer bothered me. It was at this moment though, I decided I would never, ever, berate anyone in that manner; patronising them in front of other staff and patients, should they make the unintentional mistake of borrowing my shoes.

Several years later as an anaesthetic registrar I found myself in that same situation with role reversal. I had been at the dental hospital in the morning and returned to the main hospital to anaesthetise patients on a busy urology list in the afternoon. After the pre-op visits and squeezing in some lunch, time was tight as I rushed to the changing room, only to be unable to locate my theatre shoes.

As an anaesthetic registrar on rotation for three months, you are usually given your own pair of theatre shoes which is a great treat, but you are nowhere near the higher echelons required to lay claim to a locker. There is no option but to leave ones shoes lying around at risk of being borrowed. I deducted mine had suffered this fate today. My mind flashed back to the humiliating scenario of labour ward a few years ago as I went in search of the culprit, reminding myself to keep calm and be nice!. I wandered around the theatre suite peeking through glass panels here and there, giving casual hellos to those I knew, while eyeballing everyone's feet. I knew it would not be a regular member of staff and sure enough, I spotted a medical student through the theatre window wearing my shoes.

I returned to the changing room and grabbed another, truly spare, pair of shoes like the good doctor I promised to be and returned to her theatre. I entered and discreetly tapped the girl on the shoulder, motioning her to step aside. I introduced myself and pointed out that she was wearing my shoes, explaining that normally I wouldn't mind (when actually I would) but today I had a list to get started and please could I have them back? Now, please. I had brought her these others for her to change into.

Instead of the gratitude I expected for my polite, unobtrusive handling of the situation, she scowled at me as she kicked off my shoes, rolling her eyes in exasperation that it should matter so much.'Why couldn't I just wear those others myself?' she asked.

With difficulty I remained silent and waited. Progressing from borrowed mis-matched shoes to your own personally worn in pair makes a huge difference on a daily basis. I was not giving this up so easily. Perhaps she too will come to realise this one day and will in turn pass forward some good will too.

In the following years, I notice the lengths people go to in order to deter visitors to theatre from borrowing their shoes. Some take a black marker pen and draw a skull and crossbones on the heels, other threaten with shouty words 'DO! NOT! BORROW!' but a silent warning of 'Danger. Active verrucas,' is more effective because it might just be true. The best shoe preserving technique has to be that of Mr Satish. A Professor of surgery from India, he was working in our hospital for a one year sabbatical. I noticed he wore the least popular style of theatre shoe; the neon pink plastic croc. It was hated by the girls and never, ever, worn by the men. One day I told him he should ask Sister for different shoes as more white and navy ones had recently arrived. I thought a man of his standing deserved more reserved footwear.

'No, no, no' he shook his head, 'You do not understand. I do not want different shoes. I *like* the pink ones. *I* am confident enough to wear pink shoes and besides, no-one ever borrows them!'

15. Labour Ward

Anaesthetists are introduced to obstetric anaesthesia in the labour ward and maternity theatres in the second year of training. Life is vastly different this short walk down the link corridor. The 'patients' come in to hospital without anything wrong with them. They are here to have a baby and this should be a happy experience. They should be very fit for anaesthesia if required though few anticipate any medical intervention much less an operation. Woman of child bearing age are not normally restricted by cardio-respiratory disease as seen in the older population of the main hospital. The sting in the tail of this good news is that the stakes are raised. Precisely *because* there is nothing wrong with these mothers, anything that *does* go wrong, any complication arising, takes on much greater significance compared to occurring during treatment for an illness. The risk to benefit ratio in a completely different context.

The mantra of there being not one, but two lives at stake is continual and important, yet for the anaesthetist, the importance of safe care for the mother is paramount. A mother who suffers severe morbidity or mortality during childbirth leaves a partner to cope with a newborn, his own grief as well as that of any older siblings. While thankfully rare, this is a truly tragic state of affairs. Obstetric anaesthesia is a high stakes, high speed sub specialty that I was nervously anticipating.

It is a true rite of passage to be 'on' for labour ward and this separates the proverbial men from the boys. Providing epidural pain relief on labour ward is one of the most common procedures requested and when beginning to work in any new unit, the midwives will regard you with suspicion and assume you are useless. You will gain their respect in due course when you have shown you can render their patients pain free in a swift, slick manner with minimum fuss.

I had learnt the technique of epidural insertion in other groups of patients, mostly those having hip or knee joint replacements. The key principle of sticking a thick blunt 8cm long needle into someones back to locate an area very close to their spinal cord is first and foremost to be careful, ensure absolute sterility and have the patient sit absolutely still. Compliant, rational patients understand the risks of moving, help themselves and their anaesthetist by remaining statue-like, barely daring to breathe while the needle is in their back. I was unsure how this practice would translate to a hysterical woman in the throes of labour, frantically screaming and swearing in distress at the pain and sitting on a pad, soggy from ongoing drainage of water from around the baby.

'How do you get them to sit still?' I asked my boss on my first day.

'Ah-ha! You may ask! That's the skill my dear. You'll figure it out one way or another'

Great. Very helpful. I was no further forward when the first call came. It was a typical referral to anaesthesia on labour ward by the midwife.

'Hello, Dr May here, on for anaesthetics

'EPIDURAL ROOM 2!' Phone slams down. A demand to attend rather than a request to assess the patient and provide appropriate pain relief.

As there was no opportunity for information or to form any kind of rapport on the telephone I wandered down to the control desk to find out more about the patient in room two to have some idea of the battlefield I was entering.

Her name was Joan and she was 'ideal' for me to start with I was told. It was her second baby and she was only in very early labour. She had an epidural with her first child and it was great. No pressure then. She now wanted another. In theory she should be able to sit fairly still if not yet in advanced labour and she should know something about the importance of doing so from the last time.

I entered the room, proceeding with an air of confidence I did not feel. After a quick chat I was gowned and gloved, my equipment laid out and ready. I had Joan sit up on the edge of the bed, facing the wall with her back exposed to me. I cleaned it with some antiseptic solution, warning her in advance it would feel cold.

'Aaaaaaaaaaaahhhh, you're not kidding! It's freezing!' Such melodrama did nothing for my nerves.

'Sorry. I'm sorry. Now, remember, nice and still while I'm working here'

'Aaaaaaaaaaaahhh, I can't, I think it's coming.' She said, referring to the baby.

'Now now, calm down. Take some nice deep breaths so we can get this epidural in and make you feel much better' the midwife's soothing tones had little effect.

'I'm just starting now, I'll freeze the skin and then you will feel me pushing into your back. Does that feel okay?'

'Aaaaaaaaaaaahhh, Aaaaaaaaaaaahhh'

I paused, concerned these screams were in response to the needle advancing through her skin and tissues, concerned even more by the terror and primal pain they conveyed. I was young, naiive, and horrified by this insight into early labour

I waited for a pause between the screams and gently queried 'Okay for me to continue?'

'JUST ******* WELL GET ON WITH IT! THE BABY'S COMING!'

I continued to ease the needle slowly, deeper into her back, millimetre by millimetre while the midwife reassured her the baby was not coming. Her recent examination showed her to be 4cm dilated, nowhere near the 10cm required for the baby's head to descend but it can often feel that way upon sitting up as she was now. It all sounded plausible enough. I didn't know any better.

'You're doing really well there,' I said, smiling because I knew I was doing really well too. 'Keep still just a few moments longer for me.' I could sense a change in feel from the needle meaning it was almost in the correct place. I continued to coax it forward.

'Aaaaaaaaaaaaahhh, I CAN'T! IT'S COMING! I KNOW IT'S COMING!' Without warning, she flung herself backwards towards me. Instinctively, I withdrew the needle from her back so she did not impale herself upon it, and I managed to have it out of her back before she hit the bed. 'IT'S COMING, IT'S COMING. THE BABY IS COMING! I'VE STILL GOT MY PANTS ON AND IT'S COMING'

I looked at the midwife from behind my mask and raised my eyebrows. What now?

'I'll just get some gloves on and examine you.' the calm tones a little more frenzied now.

'Aaaaaaaaaaahhh, IT'S! COMING!'

I peered between her legs. Sure enough the head was bulging out, pushing past her underwear. The midwife turned back, gloves now on, just in time to catch the baby as it was propelled out of it's mother with the force of water erupting from a blow hole.

The mother slumped in exhaustion as I took in the scene of carnage. A midwife kneeling on the floor holding the newborn, the umbilical cord with its thick rope-like appearance still attached inside the mother, making the baby look as if it had bungee jumped out. It had almost hit the floor. In the melee, an alarm was sounding and several members of staff burst into the room to help. There was blood everywhere. Lots of noise: shouts, commands, requests, instructions. The piercing screams of the mother, now naked, had given way to quieter primitive groans as she delivered the placenta. The bed was dishevelled, equipment prepared for delivery lay unused. The door opened again and the paediatric team arrived to take care of the baby. I moved my epidural trolley out of their way. Unsure of my exact role now but suspecting I no longer had one. I tidied my kit into the sharps bin feeling redundant and inadequate. I had failed. Although I had almost finished inserting the epidural before all hell broke loose I had still failed to provide the mother with the pain relief she requested to deliver her baby. I was acutely aware there was nothing I could ever do to change that or make it any better for her.

I left the room unnoticed, the chaotic scene gradually morphing into the usual pathway and protocols followed after childbirth. The frenzy was dying down. There had been a near miss but ultimately no harm had come to mother or baby: although both were a little shell shocked they remained well.

I went on to perform hundreds of epidurals in my training, becoming faster and more efficient as my experience increased. The joy of providing epidural pain relief is only spoilt by the intermittent, nature of the work predominantly in the early hours of the morning. A request for epidural analgesia could be fulfilled with the round trip to labour ward and back to bed taking only 20 minutes; in my busiest weekend I carried out 23 epidurals in a 48 hour period so you had to be quick about it.

The rewards were two fold. Expertise brought respect from the midwives and a gratifying, audible, sigh of relief when they saw it was you entering the room for their patient. The greatest reward is witnessing the transformation in patients as their pain relief kicks in. Wild women in labour who shout and swear at you, who can't or won't answer your questions, and who yell at you to get on with it, can, within 10 minutes be transformed into the most grateful, apologetic, sincere patients. Claims of hatred are replaced with declarations of love and all is forgiven.

Severe pain, like excessive alcohol, strips away our social graces, removing the lens through which we filter ourselves before presentation to the world. It lays bare our true colours complete with ugliness and failings, leaving primitive emotions on display unchecked by our conscious process of modification and masking. Above all it shows vulnerability and it is truly rewarding to be able to reassure and provide pain relief for these women at such pivotal, life changing moments.

To go back to the original question: how does one ensure these women sit still while having their epidural sited?

Unlike many other anaesthetists who strike fear into patients with risks of paralysis from the big needle, I have a much simpler technique. Believing it always better to work with the patient, I ask them to help me to help them, rather than threatening them with 'What ifs...' or 'If you don't sit still...' scenarios. So when hysteria and pain prevent compliance with instructions to sit still, I leave their back and walk around the bed to face them, calm and apologetic. I speak quietly.

'I know you are having trouble staying still for me and I understand it is really difficult. To keep it safe for you though, I can't continue with the epidural at present. I need you to stay still and I can come back at any time you feel ready to have another attempt. Just ask the midwife to call me.'

Generally, as I turn away and make for the door they realise I am going to leave without sorting out their pain relief and the panic sets in! Suddenly they ask that I stay, please, please, please stay and try again. They promise to sit still.

This time, usually they do sit perfectly still and within 20 minutes the cursing, crazed, mother ravaged with pain is transformed back to normal: face relaxed, eyes closed, a slight smile playing at her lips as she murmurs something about having a snooze.

That, is job satisfaction.

16. Urology Disaster

The urology list covered all aspects of the waterworks system and was another that we were allocated to as juniors. The thinking was that a quick look with a telescope down the urethra into the bladder was a short, minor procedure and would be straight forward. This is indeed the case but the surgical procedure being minor and straight forward does not mean the anaesthesia will be too.Not helped by the facts that the surgeon is annoyed he has been allocated a junior anaesthetist and does not make life easy for them, and the patients are precious about any procedure involving their private parts.

The patients are challenging, and fall into two main categories. The first group are old men who come for regular check ups on their prostate gland or bladder cancer (one of the few cancers that can be locally buzzed away and obliterated for long term control). These men have several heavy volumes of notes indicating multiple medical co-existing conditions being treated by a myriad of potential interacting drugs. The reassurance is that they have had the procedure before and survived the anaesthesia. Looking at the old charts will show if there were any problems and indicate in a 'recipe' type way, the ballpark doses of drugs required. Slow, careful induction of anaesthesia is the key to prevent a crash and burn of the blood pressure, quickly followed by everything else.

The second group is more problematic. These are young men who attend for circumcision or vasectomy. They are, without exception, terrified and highly anxious, and must be scraped off the ceiling with multiple meds before even beginning to put them off to sleep. Further, they try desperately to hide their anxiety. They become mono-syllabic and ask no questions, appearing nonchalant about the impending attack on their manhood. This fools no-one but the naive anaesthetist.

Looking back, I was at that blissful stage of training where I had the confidence of one who has done enough and seen enough to know what to do and how to do it but has not yet done enough and seen enough to be fully cognisant of all that can go wrong. Junior anaesthetists can be fairly blasé, verging on over confidence at times. They feel invincible and have not been around long enough to be aware of the pitfalls or witness disasters. As we mature and our experience increases, we become wise, cautious, more conservative in our practice, our aim to avoid repeating mistakes we have made and have no desire to repeat.

My first great learning experience of this type occurred in a fit, healthy young man attending for 'examination under anaesthesia'. His name was Alex and despite his calm demeanor I was ready for the anxiety to emerge and had several concoctions of drugs drawn up ready to fire into him.

He was wheeled straight into the operating theatre, the lack of separate anaesthetic rooms in modern theatres ensures fear is maximised. (Both that of the patient and the anaesthetist.) There are many good reasons for this but it ultimately means you anaesthetise patients in front of an audience of theatre nurses, surgeons and auxiliary staff. These people try to keep the noise level to a minimum and fail dismally. Hence there is significant background noise as packs are opened and the instruments clatter out, water is running while the surgeon scrubs up and a number of nurses having a variety of conversations about their holidays and what they are going to wear on Friday night. All in all it adds an additional layer of stress to a junior anaesthetist sent there to manage a challenging list, alone.

Not entirely alone though. I had an operating department practitioner (ODP) called Derek assisting me. He too, was young and felt ideally placed to reassure patients like Alex. This he did in a matey jovial way often involving high fives or good natured banter which was neither effective or professional. He treated me in the same way, but despite his personality, he was good at his job.

As I inserted the cannula into Alex's hand, Derek warned him of the impending needle.

'Small prick coming up!' he laughed as he glanced around the theatre to check everyone 'got' his clever joke. There are a number of similar phrases regularly trotted out during a urology list.

Don't balls it up.

Will-y or won't he?

Has there been a cock up?

Despite regular repetition these never fail to bring out the juvenile nature of (mostly male it has to be said) members of staff. In fact everything to do with genitalia or sex is fair game for having a laugh in urology theatre.

Derek attached the usual monitors to the Alex: leads to monitor his heart, a blood pressure cuff on his arm and a probe on his finger to measure his pulse and detect the oxygen saturation of his blood.

I gave Alex a few breaths of pure oxygen to increase the reservoir of it in his lungs and then injected a whole syringe full of anaesthetic induction agent at great speed. The drug, Propofol, can feel uncomfortable as it travels up the veins in the arm and he wriggled a little at this point, which is commonly seen.

But then he wriggled a bit more, and it was not settling. In fact, the opposite was happening. He began moving his arms up to the face mask and moaning. I fired in a second, full syringe of Propofol, and then a third, before he began to relax and allow me to take over his breathing. He was indeed anxious, a high level of adrenaline heightening his senses, requiring a much higher dose to dampen them down.

Next I inserted the laryngeal mask airway. This breathing tube does not go all the way into the lungs and fit snugly, instead it sits higher in the throat, over the vocal cords. When it is positioned correctly, the patient breathes in anaesthetic gases directly from the breathing system through this tube, and when breathing out, the expired gases are channelled through the same tube where they are analysed. This provides a vital trace of respiration and confirms the patient is alive and ventilating themselves effectively.

A sterile field is required for the operation. We moved Alex down the table to put his legs into the stirrups. They were then lifted upwards and outwards to expose his genitalia. His gown was pulled up above his waist, out of the way. His abdomen was exposed and it was fat. There was no other way to describe it. I was surprised how fat it was after being hidden well under his clothes when he arrived.

'Yep, he's a fat lad that's for sure,' the ODP confirmed, as he casually slapped the patient's stomach making it reverberate like jelly on a plate.

At this, Alex began to hiccough. My heart sank, this was all I needed. Hiccoughs are not uncommon around the start of general anaesthesia. The theories relating to why this happens include irritation of nerve controlling the diaphragm, the main muscle of breathing, or that anaesthesia may be too deep, or not deep enough! Whatever the reason, these big, loud hiccoughs upset the smooth, regular pattern of breathing and do not allow effective ventilation of the lungs. I glowered at the ODP, his matey slap on the abdomen had upset the status quo and caused problems which I then had to deal with.

I decided to watch and wait for the hiccoughs to settle on their own. Alex's blood oxygen level had reduced from 99% to 95% not yet a level to cause concern. The surgeon appeared, oblivious to my watchful state, oblivious to me it seemed! I observed the patient, his hiccoughs and monitors as the surgeon proceeded to clean the genitals by pouring freezing cold antiseptic solution liberally over the whole area.

This was intensely annoying: I'm sure he did it out of spite but more importantly, this sudden stimulation to sensitive parts of the male anatomy caused the hiccoughing patient now to buck and rear. His jaw clenched, his face turned red, and his neck veins bulged. Then came the dreaded, strained sound of air struggling to pass through a severely narrowed passage. The primitive response to stimulation greater than that which can be tolerated at the current depth of anaesthesia is to snap the vocal cords together, closing the airway. As Alex tried to breathe in, his large abdomen heaved, the sound was laboured, high pitched and drawn out before it disappeared.

It was easy to diagnose laryngospasm. Literally spasm of the voice box. Universally feared, actively avoided and heroically recounted by anaesthetists around the globe. I was in the state of fear at this moment. I watched the abdomen jerk out and in as Alex tried in vain to draw a breath against the closed cords.

The tone of pulse monitor dropped, more sinister with each beep, signifying the falling oxygen level in the patient's blood, quickly reaching a level which was of concern this time, but it did not stop. He continued to deteriorate. I was panicked. He was young and fit and healthy and must not die! I was only 26 years old and must not get struck off the medical register. My heart rate increased to rival that of the patient.

'Get me the sux and a tube now,' I yelled at the ODP. To his credit he was there with the equipment I needed immediately, although it felt as if I'd been waiting a lifetime.

As the patient turned from purple to pale, then grey, and air cannot pass in and out of the lungs, the only option is to paralyse the patient. Muscle paralysis relaxes the vocal cords and breaks laryngospasm. To prevent the scenario recurring a different tube is then placed beyond the cords into the windpipe, intubating the patient to secure the airway.

This was me, this was now, this was it. Time to put theory into practice.

The rule of optimal head, neck and pillow positioning prior to intubation was thrust aside as I gave the emergency drugs. I waited for the twitching of full paralysis to stop and removed the laryngeal mask easily, now the jaw was relaxed. I was on my tiptoes, at full stretch with my heart pounding in my ears when I was handed the metal scope. I put the blade into his mouth, using it to move the tongue aside and pulled hard. I had only a poor view of the vocal cords, but it was a view and I passed a rubber guide through the black space between them, before rail-roading the tube over it into place.

Fumbling to attach the breathing system to the tube, I squeezed the bag of oxygen into my lifeless patient. As his chest rose with each inflation I too breathed a sigh of relief. He was out of danger, we were both safe.

Gradually, the numbers on the monitors began to improve. The tone of the beeps became brighter, more optimistic and the trends reversed towards normal.

Almost in a daze, I sank down onto my stool. When I tried to pick up my pen to write the chart I realised I couldn't; my hands were shaking so much.

'Can we get on with the operation now?' The surgeon had noted the frantic activity at the head of the table and was waiting impatiently for the patient to be rendered anaesthetised, kept still, ready for surgery.

'Yes, thanks' I replied, my voice shaky too.

I abandoned the chart and concentrated on getting a grip and recovering from my first near miss. Derek, the ODP mumbled an apology for triggering the chain of events subsequent to slapping the patient's tummy.

I nodded, not trusting myself to speak. Nine months into my anaesthetic career I had witnessed first hand how quickly the tables can turn. In a matter of seconds, a fit young patient for a simple procedure had fallen prey to a series of chance events causing him to deteriorate into a critical, life threatening state that required immediate and specific action to prevent irreversible damage. Only a couple of hours before he had walked into hospital voluntarily for an investigation necessitating general anaesthesia. He was not dying from a terminal condition or being subjected to surgery as a last resort. No, when patients electively present for tests, the ratio of risk relative to benefit is much higher.

Frights like this are good (afterwards). Knowing what to do in an emergency and actually doing it are very different. I learnt from the mistakes I made that day. The anaesthetist is in charge of the patient in theatre. Even when junior to the surgeon. From that day on, I spoke up to the surgeons, even those intimidating me, asking them to wait. Wait until I was convinced of the patient's readiness for their insult. I began to voice my concerns about hiccoughs to ODPs and asked them also to wait, not touching the patient and doing as I asked, until it settled. It made me wary and cautious with each and every subsequent patient I anaesthetised, particularly the walking well.

Personal experience is the most powerful learning tool. It is not so much making the mistakes, as seeing the consequences of them and having to bail yourself out of the resulting situation that really sticks in the mind and does not dislodge in years to come. Learning through extensive exposure leads to mastery of a subject: cumulative experience informs and adjusts daily practice as a result of previous episodes, often bypassing conscious thought and deliberate decision making. This is what makes it look so easy. This is where, as juniors, we are aiming.

17. Death on the Table

I was now well aware that administering general anaesthesia transforms a walking, talking patient into an unconscious casualty who does not breathe regularly and cannot keep his tongue from obstructing his airway. It is truly a dangerous business.

Even so, it is surprisingly difficult to die when you are in an operating theatre with a competent anaesthetist present. Ready access to oxygen and adrenaline (or epinephrine to use its globally recognised name), combined with the knowledge to use these can prolong the essence of life, of heart and brain perfusion, beyond expectation. There remain times however, when mother nature and the laws of physics are too great for man (or woman) and medicine to overcome and the patient dies during an operation despite the best efforts of all involved.

The rate of death occurring under general anaesthesia is very low and occurs mostly in old, frail patients in need of emergency surgery. The first death on the operating table I witnessed was around ten months into my anaesthetic career and will always remain with me.

I was scheduled to be on another urology list, this time with one of the consultants regularly involved in my training. I will call him Dr Roberts. He was loud and self-important, with an upper class accent that I suspect was exaggerated if not entirely fictitious. But he was a great anaesthetist: a perfectionist paying great attention to detail, no sloppy standards tolerated and no prisoners taken. I held him in high regard with equal measures of respect and fear. He was a good teacher too, and endeavoured to pass on these high standards of practice to the next generation.

The list had only one patient, meaning the operation was expected to take all day. The patient was Mr Clark. He was in his sixties and was remarkably well. He lived at home with his wife where they 'looked after each other' and he walked his little dog twice each day. He had worked hard on the railways all his life and was now enjoying his retirement and travelling as a passenger to visit many places he had only passed through or been no further than the station. He had a cancerous tumour of his kidney and was having the kidney removed in an attempt to halt the spread of the disease. Overall his kidney function was unaffected: the second, healthy kidney compensating for the one which is failing. The main problem was that the tumour had started to spread aggressively. As cancers do, this tumour had grown rapidly, invading and overwhelming the normal kidney tissue, compressing it into submission as it dominated the anatomy. Such rapid growth is accompanied by pain and necessitates the development of its own blood supply, a craggy network of untidy vessels, hurriedly established to propagate the disease, lacking the ordered structure and strength of normal vessels. These new blood vessels are weak and friable: easily damaged and liable to bleed.

We anticipated significant blood loss during the procedure. Forewarned is forearmed and Dr Roberts' plan included siting additional large intravenous cannulae to pour replacement fluid and blood quickly into the circulation, and another cannula in a central neck vein to record the overall fill level of the circulation. Blood bank had given us six units of blood before the start of the operation and was standing by to provide plasma and clotting factors in addition. Maintaining normal function of the patient's body during a prolonged procedure included a urinary catheter, actively warming the patient (patients cool continually while anaesthetised) with warm fluids, a foil hat, and a hot air blanket. His temperature was monitored and his pressure areas, points of contact with the jelly mattress, were padded and regularly massaged during the operation.

Despite this, it is a good example of how a technically difficult operation may require fairly simple general anaesthesia. Apart from the tumour, Mr Clark was fairly fit. He had no heart or lung disease and didn't smoke. As the operation got underway we settled in for the duration. I was planning tea breaks and lunch. The surgery was painstakingly difficult as the surgeon meticulously dissected out the kidney without disrupting the tumour, partly to prevent bleeding but also to prevent pieces breaking free and spreading via the circulation. For this reason the renal vein, draining blood back from the kidney, towards the circulation and onward to the heart and lungs, was to be clamped. The kidneys work hard and need lots of oxygen. Therefore, they receive a large proportion of the blood pumped by the heart, approximately one quarter of it. If the heart pumps six litres of blood per minute, then 1.5 litres is allocated to the kidneys to carry out their role. If each kidney receives an equal blood supply, then there is 750 mls of blood coming and going from the kidney via the renal artery and renal vein, each and every minute. That is 12.5mls per second. That is a lot of blood.

The surgeon identified and delicately freed up the renal vein. He applied the clamp across its entire width and ratcheted it tightly closed.

The next step was to tie off the vein beyond the clamp before removing it with the kidney as a whole. The first suture was slung around the vein and pulled tight. The bleeding started almost immediately. The vein was infiltrated by tumour, newly developed since the last scan, and its wall weakened. The suture slid through the vein wall with the ease of a cheese wire.

Another suture was requested and hurriedly mounted by the scrub nurse and passed to the surgeon. Being slow and careful (very difficult when facing continual blood spillage), the surgeon placed the second suture. The same happened and the bleeding intensified. Safely at the head end of Mr Clark, we could see the surgeon's distress. 'Whenever I try to suture it, it disintegrates' he replied, his arms raised and hands upturned in disbelief and the perplexity of what to do next. What *do* you do next when the usual cure is making the problem worse?

He continued with different types of sutures, re-siting the clamp further up the vein but by then there were too many ragged breaches of the vein wall.

We actioned our plan and opened the drips on both sides, clear fluid rushing into the circulation to replace the volume of blood lost. Dr Roberts called for the blood from the fridge. The atmosphere had changed and a sinister quiet had settled, punctuated only with the short requests to the nurses by the surgeon and Dr Roberts.

After a hushed repetition in the corner confirming the blood to be correct for Mr Clark we swapped our clear fluid for two bags of blood. Then another two.

'Phone the lab and ask for six more bags as quickly as they can' instructed Dr Roberts to the staff and, to the surgeon, 'can you give us a minute to catch up?'

When the rate of blood lost exceeds our ability to match it with fluid in, we ask for a minute to catch up. The surgeon will pack the bleeding area with large swabs to temporarily dam the flow while we restore the circulating volume.

The large swabs turned quickly red and were replaced. Haemostatic gauze was called for and placed over the bleeding vein.

The blood continued to be lost. Unlike an artery, there is no muscle or elastic in the walls of veins. When an artery is cut or punctured, its response is to contract and constrict around the injury, preserving its contents. This does not happen in a vein. A hole must be stitched closed and as that strategy was not working the bleeding continued. We used all six bags of blood. A quick check revealed the blood count was only half normal. The blood from the lab still 30 minutes away.

'Get the O negative,' Dr Roberts said, 'keep pushing in clear fluid, colloid, anything, into those drips'.

I nodded realising the severity of the situation.

'How is he at your end?' the surgeon asked. This was the phrase I subsequently identified as a marker of surgical distress. It means things are not going well at their end and they are looking for reassurance that we are keeping the patient alive and asleep while they sort it out. Anaesthetists have a similar phrase they ask surgeons, 'have you got control yet?', hoping the blood loss will slow or stop any moment and the end will be in sight.

It is rare that the two phrases are heard in quick succession and generally means 'we're not winning.'

We were not winning here. The gauze was not working. We could not have our minute to catch up as the holding methods did not work and blood continued to be lost. A nurse appeared with a cloth and wiped the blood from the surgeon's visor before placing a towel on the floor to prevent him slipping on the blood now accumulating on the floor, the drapes long since saturated. I had been instructed to make up an adrenaline syringe which was now being pumped into the patient. Adrenaline restores blood pressure when the circulation is under filled and demands the heart work harder to compensate. The rate was increased further and further until any effect could be seen and I could feel my own adrenaline levels increase in proportion; the typical 'flight or fright' response that arms us to face or flee from danger and threat had kicked in. The surgeons continued to battle: more stitches, more swabs, more hands in Mr Clark's abdomen, more blood, more instruments, more tension and more failure.

I brought more potent syringe jets of adrenaline from the resuscitation trolley and began to administer large boluses at a time. Dr Roberts noticed and nodded. The ODP continued to pressurise the fluids and change the bags when empty. The used bags were thrown into a pile on the floor: they would be counted and documented later. The numbers on our screen were dropping despite throwing everything there was at, what could now only be described as exsanguination. The screen was flashing, the monitor's alarms activated to remind us: blood pressure low, no peripheral perfusion,

The carbon dioxide trace dwindled. This, the one trace that confirms the patient is alive and well was far from its normal value. Mr Clark's colour had changed. He was grey and his face looked waxy, signifying its lack of perfusion as blood was preferentially directed only where strictly necessary, the brain and the heart. The bleeding continued to out pace us all.. With no blood perfusing the coronary arteries, no oxygen is delivered to the heart muscle and its synchrony is lost. The fibres of the heart muscle reach firing level randomly, chaotically, ineffectively and the circulation lost, culminating in cardiac arrest.

Dr Roberts commenced cardiac compressions. We all knew this was futile; cardiac arrest being only a symptom rather than the cause of the true problem. We had not managed to control the bleeding problem in the last 30 minutes and we were not going to do so now. The purpose was to display the stage of deterioration we had now reached and to allow a consensus opinion to be confirmed: to continue would be futile. It was time to stop.

The surgeon left the operating table, snapping his gloves off he flung them to the floor, ripping off his gown and slamming it into the bin as the door to the scrub room banged shut. Momentary silence descended upon the theatre team before we all seemed to feel the same need to be occupied purposefully. I silenced the alarms on the monitors and closed the drips, unsure of protocol in this situation. The surgeon's assistant proceeded to close the abdomen with thick, coarse sutures placed without precision or planning, required only to hold the two skin edges together.

Dr Roberts turned off the anaesthetic gases and finally, having no choice, he turned off the ventilator. I felt a morbid finality, never before experienced. It was over. The procedure, the anaesthetic, the life. Mr Clark's life was now undisputedly over and my overriding thought at that moment was not for Mr Clark, nor his wife. It was not for the surgeon or Dr Roberts. It was for me. I was glad I was not in charge. Glad for once that I was a trainee having responsibility only to learn, not yet having to take responsibility for big decisions or the outcomes that followed. No-one had done anything wrong or forgotten any vital step yet the patient had died. I was not ready to have that weight on my shoulders.

It would be 14 years later that I found myself in charge of a similar case and the weight of the outcome would sit heavily on my shoulders. By then I had experience and confidence yet still, it did not sit comfortably and I doubt it ever does. With modern medicine advancing rapidly there is a terrible feeling of redundancy, of futility when all that we have is not enough and the patient dies mid procedure.

Many weeks later Dr Roberts was able to discuss this whole event in lighter terms. The situation was not any lighter as time passed but this is the medics' way of coping. To joke and dismiss stressful events as par for the course allows difficulties to be aired and for others to empathise and reassure that they too, would have done the same (while thanking their lucky stars it was not them). Dr Roberts' conversation to me now was philosophical.

'That's why I get paid the big bucks. I don't earn my money doing the routine, regular work week in and week out. I earn it from the big decisions, the bad outcomes, by taking responsibility.' he said, 'you know, massive haemorrhage is nothing to be afraid of as an anaesthetist. All you have to do is keep pouring in the blood, the fluid, the clotting factors, then more blood more fluid and more clotting factors until the surgeon stops the bleeding. Think of it as a bath, you keep filling it up while he figures out how to put the plug in.'

The surgeon anaesthetist cooperative ethos of the event was long gone and normal banter, depicting clever anaesthetists and stupid surgeons was back.

'Besides,' he continued, 'think about it: all bleeding stops eventually.'

18. Pre-operative Visiting

It was several weeks later when I worked with Dr Roberts again on that same list, and it was equally memorable. One of the key learning situations in anaesthesia is visiting the patients before their operation. It benefits both the patient and the doctor: patients have an opportunity to ask questions, and familiarity with the plan reduces their anxiety. The doctor can find out about medical problems the patient has and make a plan for anaesthesia and pain relief in light of this knowledge. Premedication can be prescribed if required and there is still an over night to come up with a plan if you have uncovered something challenging. The responsibility for seeing the patients pre-operatively lies with the senior anaesthetist responsible for the list, but as the trainee, I was expected to see the patients for my own learning.

The day before I had finished late and felt tired. In truth, I couldn't be bothered to trudge to the ward to see this one patient for the following day; the plan would be as before, plan for bleeding, extra lines and so on, and this man was younger and I assumed he wouldn't have much else wrong with him. I left the hospital planning to arrive early the next day to say a quick 'hello' to him before he went to theatre. This was vitally important as the consultant would make a show of introducing me in the anaesthetic room.

'And you've met Dr May?' he would enquire of the patient as he indicated me.

Heaven help you if you hadn't seen the patient, or he failed to recognise you now dressed up in theatre garb complete with paper hat.

'Yes, we met up on the ward,' I would interject, passing the first test of the day and increasing the chance of it being pleasant thereafter. Even better was to greet the patient arriving in the anaesthetic room with a smile of recognition and a greeting of 'Nice to see you again Mr Patient, did you get much sleep last night?' but this was not always possible and bluffing was a high risk strategy.

Again, this day there was only one patient for a major procedure. Of course I slept in, arrived later than planned, dashed to the ward just in time to see the theatre porters and my patient disappear from sight as the lift doors closed. I ran back down the stairs to catch the patient in theatre reception. This necessitated getting changed into theatre clothes but thankfully, I was now pretty quick at this!

I emerged from the changing room and the patient was nowhere to be seen. It was a toss up between waiting to see the patient and being late to the anaesthetic room making my absence conspicuous and meaning Dr Roberts would be drawing up all the drugs himself.

I decided to go straight to the anaesthetic room and see how things panned out as regards meeting the patient. Dr Roberts was not there so I began to prepare the drugs with a sigh of relief: for all he knew I could have been here for ages! Then the door swung open.

'Good morning Ellie.' he boomed, full of self importance. 'What did you make of this chap's story then?' he was straight to the point. Thinking honesty to be the best policy and knowing that Dr Roberts liked me, I looked him in the eye and confessed I had not seen the patient pre-operatively.

'How can you expect to plan their anaesthetic if you know nothing about them?' Still very conversational, yet before I could fight my corner he continued 'off you go then.'

I looked at him, puzzled.

'There's no point to you being here if you know nothing about what's going on, what we're going to do and why we're doing it. Off you go.'

He shooed me away as if I were a nuisance, a mere irritation to him.

At first I could not move, I was rooted to the spot, stunned by his command and at sea as to what I should do. Then I turned on autopilot and did the walk of shame out of theatre, shocked beyond tears (until I reached the changing rooms anyway). I was humiliated, annoyed and frustrated. Annoyed at being sent away, annoyed at not defending myself, annoyed at the patient for leaving the ward just as I'd got there. There was no joy in an unexpected day off. It stretched ahead and I wondered how I would fill it.

I got changed back again, my clothes still warm and once I decided I was in a fit state to leave the changing room, I went to that universal safe haven where trainee doctors can lick their battle wounds; the secretaries' office. Here I was guaranteed tea and biscuits along with sympathy and gentle agreements that yes, I was in the right and whatever has happened was unjust and no, I did not deserve it.

After an hour or so of chat I felt better and went home to spend the rest of the day feeling depressed, eating cake and watching meaningless day time television. If nothing else I like to think I learn from my errors and the next week I was scheduled for the same list with the same consultant. Full of impending doom, I dragged myself to the ward the night before, to see the patients. There were 10 patients on the list for the following day. All for regular check ups and minor procedures yet had case-notes extending to several volumes. The previous anaesthetic charts completed by Dr Roberts often stated simply 'Known to me' instead of the extended version of the medical history detailing their multiple medical problems.

Unfortunately, the patients were not known to me and I spent over three hours seeing them, making sure I could remember something about each of them. (This was harder than it sounds as they were all men aged between 60 and 80 years of age, with long term bladder problems and an assortment of high blood pressure, angina, chronic bronchitis and diabetes).

I arrived home, exhausted at 9 pm to find the light flashing on my answering machine. I pressed play and did not expect to hear 'Message from Dr Roberts for Dr May...'. My heart sank. What had I done now? His formal, pompous tones continued, filling my small room with his '...profuse thanks for seeing all the patients this evening' and stating that 'he really appreciated it as had finished late himself'. Listening almost brought a lump to my throat: a mixture of relief and pride at his praise, coming in contrast to the shame of the week before and combined with the chronic tiredness that makes many junior doctors overly emotional. With his exacting standards he was hard to please but, it had to be said, he was fair.

The next morning I skipped into work. I was no longer afraid of the day in theatre ahead. Knowing I was starting the day with the upper hand rather than slinking back with my tail between my legs had turned my world the right way up again.

I now explain to trainees who have failed to see my patients pre-operatively why it is important to do so. I don't believe in humiliating them, and this method of teaching is no longer common in medicine. However, I think my approach has far less impact upon trainees. It is too touchy feely, politically correct and does not serve as the stark lesson in taking responsibility for your patients, as I received and ultimately benefitted from.

19. Collapse of Obstetrician

Professionalism is not always reciprocated and it may be nothing at all to do with what grade you are and everything to do with the simple unpleasant demeanour of the surgeon. Dr Taylor was one such obstetrician.

Anaesthetising ladies to deliver their babies by Caesarean section is a pleasant, happy experience, especially in the elective setting when there are no worries about the fetal well being nor any rush to expedite delivery. But as usual, the surgeon you are working with can make or break the day. This day, it was broken beyond repair.

Dr Taylor had worked in the delivery suite for about 30 years. I had worked there too for the last seven of them, on a regular basis. I knew I had worked with him many times before so cannot fathom how he could not have that same recollection and he maintained his aloof nature and pretended to be unaware of my existence. Not only did he not know my name, he never said 'Good morning', never gave a nod of acknowledgment when passing within six inches of me in the corridor. He seemed to look straight through me and appeared surprised if I ever spoke, as if wondering where the noise had come from. Weird, yes but I tried not to take it personally. It didn't matter to me if he said hello or not but it did make it rather odd when I was the anaesthetist for his morning operations and he did not communicate with me in any way.

During any surgical procedure communication between the surgeon and anaesthetist is vital, but especially when the patient is awake and alert though numb, as for Caesarean section. The communication is often implicit to prevent undue anxiety in the mother; a brief nod to give a second dose of oxytocin if the uterus does not contract well following delivery of the placenta. This alerts me to an increased blood loss, as does his asking for the suction to be changed. Information carries the other way when I say loudly to the patient 'I'm giving you a little oxygen through this mask now and will put a drip into your other hand too'. These deviations from routine means I am not 100% happy with the state of the patient so please get on and finish the operation quickly.

The first patient, to be honest, was not the brightest. This was her second Caesarean section and she just wanted to 'Ger it owt', while being 'knocked owt o' it'. I made the case for regional anaesthesia, where she could be awake but numb for her delivery and she agreed to this on the understanding that she 'Wood no feel owt'.

The operation proceeded as expected. No communication across the blood brain barrier, that drape that separates the surgical field from the anaesthetist, but things were going well so it didn't matter too much. There had been slight concern about on-going bleeding but Dr Taylor now appeared happy (figuratively speaking) or at least satisfied that it was not problematic and had closed the wound. He mumbled to the patient that he was going to lift her legs to 'check for bleeding down below' and I duly translated to her what was about to happen despite this being way too much information that she did not need to know.

'Down below' a series of swabs were inserted and removed, each coming out soaked in blood. Several more were used but the result was always the same. Dr Taylor turned to the patient to say he was going to re-open her abdomen after all, to find the source of the bleeding. She expressed her annoyance that the procedure was not yet over, having taken longer than she remembered and urged him to 'ger oan wi-it'.

Before doing so Dr Taylor wanted to have one more look down below. With the patients legs splayed out and held up, he bent his head between her knees to reassess the bleeding.

'Swab,' he stuck his hand out and the nurse placed the required swab into his hand.

He inserted it into the patient and again observed, watching and waiting before making his final decision. While hunched over, looking up between the patients legs, he then appeared to lean in further, as if to get a better look. It looked slightly inappropriate and seemed a bit odd, but then he *was* a bit odd. As the seconds passed and he remained still, silent. Puzzled, questioning looks passed between me, the scrub nurse and Dr Taylors junior assistant, each of us wondering what was going on.

'What's he doing down there?' I mouthed and pointed.

They both shrugged. We continued to observe as Dr Taylor moved from peering closely, to allowing his forehead to rest on the patient's leg! More looks were exchanged. This really was bizarre. As his body appeared to relax and slump further between the legs of the patient we realised Dr Taylor was unconscious. He had collapsed and was unresponsive to his name being called and his arm being shaken.

After such a prolonged, passive pause, we sprung into action. Lifting Dr Taylor up and off the patient we laid him on the floor inadvertently within view of the patient. His glasses had snapped and he looked grey and sweaty. Someone ran to the phone to call for a replacement obstetrician and anaesthetist. I was torn between monitoring and stabilising my newly delivered, possibly still bleeding patient, or tending to my newest casualty on the floor. I glanced at them both.

'Y'd best ger 'im saw-hed, 'ee looks no right'. She read my mind. She was right, he looked awful. As she watched I opened his mouth, trying to ignore his foul breath and poor dentition, and slipped an airway over his tongue to keep it clear of his throat. Next I attached an oxygen mask to his face. It misted up intermittently confirming he was still breathing. Thank goodness: no mouth to mouth required. Much to the dismay of some, he still had a pulse too. I checked for signs of incontinence, suggestive of a seizure, but his trousers were dry. Nobody knew anything about his medical history or whether he had been feeling unwell that day. I looked around for some monitoring to attach to him now, but there was no spare kit immediately to hand.

I asked for someone to get another set of chest leads and, after what seemed like an age, I was handed a set of ECG leads for his heart and a pulse oximeter for his oxygen level. It felt strangely amusing, taking the scissors to cut open his theatre top, right down the middle the way they do on television! Even worse, I had to find an area of non-hairy skin to put the sticky dots onto (ugh!). We were still on the floor and when a trolley was brought in there was no obvious way to get him onto it. It was not like the ambulance trolleys that go lower as well as higher.

It took six of us. Randomly, we each held the body part of Dr Taylor closest to us. We man-handled him up onto the trolley. A grown man, unconscious, is seriously heavy. At least his vital observations looked ok. His pulse and blood pressure were on the low side so I stuck an intravenous cannula into his arm, measured his blood sugar and got some fluids running. My plan was to wheel him around to casualty and let them deal with him but I could not yet leave the potentially bleeding lady on the operating table.

Replacement colleagues for me and my casualty arrived. They looked at the situation, hardly believing their eyes. It did look and sound fantastical. As I explained to the anaesthetist the probability that the lady was bleeding internally and needed re-opened, he took in the pulse and blood pressure displayed and remarked that she was not showing any signs of blood loss, if anything the heart rate was low.

Only when I followed the leads from the monitor did I realise that, in the panic, a well meaning auxiliary nurse had taken the monitoring equipment from the new mother and given it to me to attach to our medical casualty. Same with the pulse probe. Our original patient was, in fact, unmonitored and could be suffering no end of sequelae from occult blood loss, as we remained blissfully unaware.

Once the mistake was recognised the monitoring was quickly corrected and I left theatre to wheel my colleague through the hospital to the emergency department. They were somewhat bemused to be presented with a monitored patient, treatment underway, entering from the hospital side rather than the main doors.

Dr Taylor was beginning to regain consciousness by this point so I left swiftly lest he realise it was me who had cut his top off!

I returned to the maternity department, musing over the bizarre events of the morning. I was relieved to discover my new mother and baby were both doing well and there had been no on-going bleeding to worry about.

A few hours later I telephoned around to casualty for any news. Dr Taylor had been transferred to coronary care. The blood tests and heart tracings confirmed he had suffered a heart attack. It could not have happened to a nicer person. In the days to come he recovered well enough to be discharged home.

He returned to work a few months later and I passed him once or twice in the corridor. The first time, after 'the event', I recognised him at the opposite end of the corridor and as we walked towards one another I was anxious about what to say or do, and embarrassed about what he might remember from his collapse. I decided I would hide behind professionalism. I would bear no grudge and put his personality and social failings firmly behind me. I would accept his thanks graciously before politely moving on.

We were now only a few feet apart. I glanced up to make eye contact. Dr Taylor continued to stare straight ahead, seemingly fixated upon some vague point in the distance. As our paths grew closer still, he was not slowing down. He was not moving to the middle of the corridor in preparation for any greeting.

He walked straight past me!

Not a flicker of recognition or even a nod of vague acquaintance to a colleague we are aware of but whom we do not know. It seemed I was invisible-again.

I was speechless at first. Then indignant. A little offended. Had I not literally saved his life that day? And now he hadn't afforded me even the briefest courtesy (not to mention flowers, chocolates, champagne and a thank you card for my portfolio)? Then I saw the funny side and burst out laughing. He was just a grumpy old man who had been unwell. He had no interest in anyone or anything. He needed to retire, and a few short months later, he did just that and has never been seen since.

20. Expensive Scare

The dark side of anaesthesia, the juxtaposition of life and death, is more often seen in the intensive care unit. My first rotation to intensive care was during my second year of anaesthetic training. It was a big step.

Now I was the first port of call for casualty, ward referrals, admissions from theatre and I carried the cardiac arrest bleep which, surprisingly, was the least stressful aspect! (At a cardiac arrest there is a set protocol for managing the situation, of which everyone involved is aware. The diagnosis is simple and management is standard.)

On my first day I was told the two golden rules of intensive care. The first states that if the diagnosis is unknown, the patient will not get better. This is almost always true. Medicine and machines can support failing systems in the body to maintain an internal equilibrium, but usually, a patient's demise has been precipitated by an acute, intercurrent illness: an infection, an inflammatory process, a malignant process, for example. Whatever the cause, it must be accurately diagnosed and the appropriate, specific therapy given, if the patient is to recover. The intensive care buys time, props up the body, while this diagnosis is figured out and the treatment instituted. Random therapy aimed at treating the *signs* of the illness is merely tinkering around the edges and will not address the root cause.

The second rule is that when there has been no change in a patient's condition since the day before, the patient is actually worse. This is because despite a further 24 hours of around the clock intensive care, there has been no improvement. To be 'stable' is not always a good thing.

Intensive care, or expensive scare as it is known, is largely the domain of the anaesthetists. We run it during the day and man it 24/7.

I quickly realised I didn't like working on intensive care. It epitomises all that I did not want in a medical career namely continuity of care, prolonged periods of care for patients and chronic illnesses that improve in a two steps forward one step backwards fashion, if at all. While as a junior doctor, I routinely saw patients on the wards approach their end of life; whatever had necessitated their admission to hospital was to be their last illness. We all knew this and accepted it: the doctors, the nurses, the family and commonly the patient too. The consultant would decree the extent of the on-going care to be provided and decided which interventions would and would not be appropriate. As I progressed through training in anaesthesia, this sensible culture changed and currently it seems that no-one is allowed to die in hospital unless they have been referred to intensive care, assessed by intensive care and ultimately refused intensive care due to fact that they are dying. Medics around the hospital appear reluctant to make this call now, probably due to a combined relative lack of experience, being so busy they see this as something they can delegate, the increased expectations of the 'service users' with an over-arching fear of complaint or legal action being taken if it is perceived that not 'everything was done'.

When patients die it is always sad for some people. As a doctor, and an anaesthetist it is awful if 'your' patient dies but thankfully we do not know them long enough to know them well, as this makes it easier to feel detached. Deaths in intensive care are particularly sad and memorable but are an inherent part of this job. One quarter of patients admitted to intensive care die there and during the course of the illness, staff including doctors and nurses, come to know the patient and their relatives and are that much closer. The first death that remains with me is that of Susan and she died on this, my first exposure to intensive care.

Susan was 17 years old. Young, fit and previously healthy, as many are, before the catastrophic event precipitating their admission to intensive care. She had delivered a baby girl the night before, four weeks early due to severe pre-eclampsia. This disorder arises from the placenta and presents in the mother as dangerously high blood pressure and leaky blood vessels causing protein loss. There is, at times dramatic, swelling of the tissues and breathlessness as fluid collects in the lungs. There are varying degrees of severity and patients respond to treatment with varying degrees of success.

The ultimate treatment is to remove the placenta, the source, by delivering the baby even if premature. Even then, the pathological process can continue to get worse before it gets better, as happened to Susan and she rapidly developed multi-organ system failure.

She was brought to the intensive care unit where machines and drugs took over the role of her body's failing systems, aiming to ensure as near normal function of each continued while giving her defenses a chance to battle the illness and repair the damage.

But she had no chance.

Her young body was overwhelmed with rampant disease which showed no sign of abating. During the 12 hours following her admission, her organs failed one by one until she was swollen, bleeding spontaneously around puncture sites and no longer responding to the drugs that kept her alive.

I looked at her boyfriend who had been recontacted as Susan deteriorated. Would he come and look after the baby? A baby he didn't know he had. A baby he didn't know if he wanted. To say he was shell shocked would be an understatement.

He was 18 years old and was instantly dropped into this very different world. He sat at the bedside seeing a girl he once cared for but no longer recognised. There, he met her parents for the first time and they engaged in awkward conversation for which there is no protocol.

When Susan died I looked at him: bewildered, unsure, holding his new daughter awkwardly. I wondered how nature could be so cruel as to take a mother without concern for her newborn child? To take a young daughter without concern for her parents?

The paths of so many lives changed for ever in such a tragic way that day. I had never felt so sad in all my 25 years.

21. And Darker Still

It is well recognised that anaesthesia is a high risk specialty for doctors as well as patients. The defense union fees are significant and cover costs arising when decisions are taken which contribute to poor outcomes for patients. They do nothing to protect the anaesthetist from exposure to the risks and consequences of mental illness, suicide or addiction, either in friends, colleagues or themselves.

Why should anaesthetists be more vulnerable than doctors in other specialities to the risk of suicide? There are many factors.

Anaesthesia is a service specialty. From a very junior age and stage of training you find yourself working alone. A junior anaesthetist can safely go on call knowing only one or two techniques to put people to sleep for a variety of operations. Surgeons, in contrast, have to be able to do many different operations before they can work independently. Thus there is usually a surgical *team*, consisting of doctors of varying grades, each of whom request the help of a senior when things progress beyond their own competence. They are each part of this team.

Similarly in the medical wards, the ward round will be led by the consultant physician accompanied by his entourage of juniors, trainees and medical students. It is usual for them to go for coffee as a team when the round is finished. Although cliched, this allows bonding and an increased knowledge of colleagues beyond the walls of the hospital. Junior doctors are well supported by seniors. They are all part of the same team.

In contrast, anaesthetists working in the operating theatre usually do so alone, without the presence of any other anaesthetists. There is no anaesthesia team. We bear the burden of responsibility alone and can easily become isolated. Of course, this type of working may attract those to this specialty who are introverted and prefer working alone. But there are equal numbers of loud, gregarious extroverts in anaesthesia too.

There is a great deal of stress in anaesthesia. Some is obvious and predictable: we render patients unconscious and unable to breathe without assistance, we aim to pour blood into a patient more quickly than the surgeon is spilling it, but many stressors are less obvious and boil down to a lack of control.

We lack control in many respects: control of our workload, control of our working hours, and control of the patients. Anaesthesia is a service specialty, provided where it is required.

These are aspects of day to day working we do not control. All these examples and more are decided by surgeons, time and space in theatre, porters on their lunch break and so on. We respond to the needs of surgeons and their patients are presented to us as their circumstances dictate. We don't initiate our own plans of treatment because no patient comes into hospital with the purpose of having an anaesthetic. They come for an operation, or with an illness or an accident requiring treatment. Unlike surgeons, we do not have the luxury of choosing our patients. This lack of control and loss of part of the autonomy afforded to doctors is undoubtedly stressful.

Such background daily stress can be added to by acute illness, by a medico legal investigation, by a personal tragedy, and this may result in stress reaching an intolerable level. The level of stress exceeds the individual's capacity to deal with it. When this happens the sufferer has limited options. Ask for help and risk looking weak and 'not up to the job' or find another way to bring it to a halt.

I know two colleagues who have committed suicide.

One colleague was very senior to me and I didn't know him particularly well. Another, however was different. I'll call her Sarah.

Sarah was one of us. Together we were four senior house officers in our mid to late twenties, manning the intensive care unit 24 hours a day, seven days a week. It was a one night in four rota. The intensive care had nine beds which meant it was a large and busy unit. It was an all encompassing, exhausting job: I was either at work, sleeping or about to return to work. My free time was typified by being too physically tired to do any exercise, too mentally tired to do anything other than watch television, yet not tired enough to sleep. I would do without milk at home rather than be bothered to go and buy some. Pre mobile phones any communication with family and friends fell away, many friends working similar rotas too.

We often remarked the overnights were a combination of Russian roulette and 'there by the grace of god go us', as we arrived each morning to hear about the emergencies and disasters of the preceding night shift. I was not alone in regularly thinking 'That sounds awful, I'm glad I wasn't on last night.' But we knew it could easily have been any one of us. The stakes were raised if anyone asked you to swap a shift. Would you be trading a potentially quiet night for a career threatening catastrophe?

When Sarah took her own life we all had to deal with it. Quite literally.

Sarah, like the majority of anaesthetists who commit suicide, did so using anaesthetic drugs. The reasons are increased availability and knowledge of how these drugs work meaning they can be used to be rapidly fatal. Sarah used local anaesthetic drugs rather than the more common general anaesthetic drugs. She was very clever and had planned it well. Local anaesthetics are not controlled drugs and are not drugs of abuse. There is no high, no addiction, no point in taking them illicitly. When injected into tissues they make nerve endings go numb and are used regularly by dentists as well as anaesthetists. They are not kept in locked cupboards in hospitals and in our theatres they were readily available on trolleys for epidurals and other local anaesthetic techniques, where a part of the body is numbed rather than the patient being rendered unconscious.

This may seem to make them safe but the opposite is true. Local anaesthetics can be safely injected into the tissues around the nerves to be blocked. They are incredibly dangerous when injected directly into the circulation. When this happens the drug clings to heart muscle cells almost irreversibly, and stops the heart from beating.

One evening, Sarah had gone to the furthest end of the theatre suite and into an anaesthetic room that was deserted. She drew up a syringe of local anaesthetic and while fully conscious deliberately injected this directly into a vein in her arm.

Her heart would have stopped almost instantly.

Some time passed before Sarah was found. Too long. She was cold and remained pulseless. Despite this, active resuscitation was initiated. Although she never regained consciousness, the return of a pulse, a sign of circulation, was achieved. Sarah was transferred to the very same intensive care unit as she and the remaining three of us worked. She received no sedation yet did not awaken.She was diagnosed brain dead and died three days later.

Those three days were amongst the worst of my life.

There was distress all around. Having a colleague as a patient is very stressful under 'normal' circumstances, when all is routine and their care facilitates recovery following an accident or illness. When overlain with tragic events, distraught parents, and the guilt we were all feeling, it became unbearable. When a colleague admits a patient to intensive care you think how easily it could have been you on call that night, having to deal with it. This time it felt as if it really could have been any of us, on either side of the doctor-patient interaction.

Many major traumatic events are known to leave those who witnessed it with survivor guilt and post traumatic stress disorder. We were no different. Could we have seen it coming? Should we have seen it coming? Could we have prevented it? How did we not notice things had become so bad for Sarah that she could see no other way out than to take her own life? Had she hid her true feelings well or were we just bad colleagues more concerned with ourselves?

We were reluctant to acknowledge a sense of relief when she died after those three long days, when we could pack the whole episode away somewhere in a corner of our brain and close our minds to it.

Anaesthetists are human beings too and we can be blasé. It is in part a coping mechanism, a way to bring difficult events into conversation with others and a way to relate our working lives to everyday life. We are not the only ones who say 'Oh well, no one died' as we try to put events into perspective. This time it was different. This time someone had died. We will never forget her.

22. Failure to Wake up

As many observe and comment upon (often in a sarcastic manner), putting patients off to sleep is pretty straight forward: little clear syringe, big white syringe, medium clear syringe. This is in part true, but waking them up at the other end of the operation is somewhat more tricky. It is easily forgotten that there are as many complications when waking patients up as there are when putting them off to sleep.

The propensity for problems at the end of the operation is compounded by a theatre team for whom the operation is over. Now chatting, laughing, washing the floor and passing the mop over your feet to encourage you to get on with it, as you await patiently to allow the patient to emerge smoothly. Further, it is difficult to predict the exact moment the patient will wake up: it could be in a few seconds or several minutes but whenever it is, you must be vigilant and ready for it. This contrasts with induction of anaesthesia where the patients go off to sleep only when the anaesthetist decides.

I was around 14 months into my training when I had a patient who not so much didn't wake up, but didn't wake up as I expected.

I was working in a coastal town at the time and many of the patients were holiday makers. Mr Grant was one such patient. After a glorious day out on a boat trip, he had lost his balance stepping off the boat and twisted his ankle. On inspection, the ankle was clearly broken and required an operation to fix it so he was admitted to hospital. On admission to the ward his blood pressure was checked as a matter of routine and found to be very high. Worryingly high in fact.

On questioning Mr Grant was unaware he had high blood pressure. He hadn't seen a doctor in years, didn't take any medicines, and had no recollection of when his blood pressure was last checked. The medical doctors in the hospital were asked to see him and they advised starting him on medication to control his blood pressure. Its effect would wear on gradually over the next few days and lower his blood pressure. He would need to remain on it, or similar medication, for the rest of his life.

It was a lot for a 70 year old man, in a strange place with a painful injury while on holiday to comprehend. By now the fractured ankle had swollen to twice its size and the operation was delayed to wait for this to subside. This was no bad thing as it allowed some time to gain some control over his blood pressure.

Untreated high blood pressure is dangerous peri-operatively, increasing the risk of stroke and heart attacks.

His wife spent her time at the hospital too, dividing her time between his bedside and the coffee shop downstairs. She kept his bedside locker well supplied with bananas and grapes, they were on holiday after all. The get well soon cards began to roll in, among them his favourite, a hand drawn self portrait of his granddaughter with a speech bubble that shouted 'Come Home Soon Grandad!'

It was my day on call when he came to theatre around 9pm (a 24 hour day). There can be dangerous surges in blood pressure at induction of general anaesthesia: it can plummet as the drugs are given then soar well above normal as the breathing tube is placed into the windpipe. I knew this and was careful to give a large enough dose of a supplementary drug to attenuate these responses and aim to keep the blood pressure as steady as possible.

It all went smoothly, very smoothly, and I was congratulating myself on the neatness and uniformity of my chart, showing the blood pressure and heart rate had hardly budged throughout the procedure. In fact, I had given only a little morphine as pain relief as he had shown no signs of requiring it. It made a gratifying change from a chart depicting the course of the blood pressure more akin to a

Himalayan mountain range with random ups and downs throughout. This was a job well done.

It was time to wake him up and I switched off the gas and cleared the back of his throat with the suction tube. He didn't cough or gag at this which is always good. Coughing prevents the smooth return of regular breathing but the absence of a cough did not ring any alarm bells for me. I surmised he must be more deeply anaesthetised than I expected, hence his lack of response to the stimulation. I explained to the theatre staff, impatient as ever, that he may be a while waking up. It is common for us juniors to find this at the end of a case. So desperate are we to ensure a patient is not aware under anaesthesia we tend to err on the side of caution and give too much gas rather than too little. Theatres are used to delays like this but not particularly understanding. It *is* a pain having to wait and a lot of muttering followed to the effect that I should 'Just pull the tube out and get on with it' as they have seen many before me do. I waited as the ventilator continued to inflate the lungs, the chest moving up and down, removing the anaesthetic gas breath by breath. Another reason for being slow to wake up is being given too much morphine. This is not a big problem and it means the patient is very comfortable when he does wake up, but Mr Grant had not had too much morphine. He had barely had half of the dose I had prepared for him: his stable observations implied he was not in pain.

After about 15 minutes he began to show signs of waking up. I watched as he made a few gasps and gagged on the tube once or twice. I waited for him to settle down and breath regularly, effectively, but this did not seem to be happening and the gagging and coughing continued as his face grew red and his eyes began to tear.

I got 'the twitcher' out, the machine to assess the degree of muscle paralysis. I double checked the muscle relaxant had worn off completely, ensuring the muscles of breathing could work normally. With this confirmed, the signs still did not improve and he continued to cough and gag but did not open his eyes nor obey commands. It was not normal and Mr Grant's distress was evident by his deep purple hue and bulging neck veins. His blood pressure now was far from stable.

Instinctively I put him back to sleep to restore some calm and control in the first instance. I took over his breathing once again but had no idea what was going on, so I called for help. There was a registrar over on the maternity unit who agreed to come over to help me.

While we awaited his arrival, I checked Mr Grant's blood glucose and temperature. When low, both can cause coma, but both tests gave normal results. I looked in his eyes to find his pupils were small and equal, a reassuring sign.

Dr Atul arrived to help me. I was glad to have him there to share the burden. I recounted the story so far and his opinion was that Mr Grant had not had enough pain relief. He administered a large bolus of morphine and also some anti-anxiety medicine, before once again switching off the gas and awakening the patient.

All eyes were fixed on Mr Grant as he once again began to awaken. He coughed. He held his breath. He bucked on the tube and turned purple. It looked awful. It was exactly the same as before. I was glad in a way that Dr Atul could witness it for himself rather than simply take my word for it. He too was puzzled, unsure what was going on, but he knew what to do.

While I put Mr Grant back to sleep yet again, my colleague telephoned intensive care and arranged for Mr Grant to be admitted, to be kept sedated overnight and the situation to be reviewed by the consultant in the morning. Time remains a great healer. We packaged Mr Grant onto a trolley and wheeled him upstairs for observation overnight.

The next day it was after 5pm before I made my way up to intensive care to find out what had happened to Mr Grant that day. I was sure the consultant would have found a simple explanation for his symptoms the night before and would have him awake and right as rain by now.

I entered the unit and saw Mr Grant looking pretty much the same as when I had left him here the night before. I said hello to Mrs Grant and went to find the consultant. I saw him at the desk. As I walked over he looked up at me, grim faced.

'I was coming to look for you,' he said, 'Mr Grant.'

'Yes, what was wrong with him?' I began to feel uneasy.

'We couldn't get the tube out this morning either. He wouldn't wake up so we took him for a CT scan of his head. Massive haemorrhage, lots of blood all over his brain. No hope of any recovery. Just giving Mrs Grant some time to let the news sink in before we withdraw.'

Withdraw treatment?

I was stunned and felt physically sick. I had so many questions yet I was lost for words. Was it because of his blood pressure? Was it my fault? Was I in trouble? Had I caused his inevitable death?

'I phoned the coroner,' he continued. 'You're lucky you gave some additional opioid at the start. He seemed happy enough you had made some effort to prevent a surge in blood pressure causing him to stroke out. He's not taking the case.'

Oh good. Oh God. I felt awful. I felt awful for poor Mr Grant, upset for his wife, upset at the whole series of events. Selfishly, while I was horrified to have caused the catastrophe, I was relieved I was not being held to account for it. Rather, it was one of those bad things that happen to good people, which seems so trite when it relates to an individual.

After hearing this news, I sat with Mrs Grant for a while. I held her hand but we didn't speak. I think she understood exactly what had happened and had the grace not to vent her anger and grief towards me. I had done my best yet I left knowing the life support machine was to be turned off. There was to be no recovery.

Mr Grant died later that day. His wife packed his things and left for the train station to head back home.I said goodbye knowing I would never see her again, knowing it would be some time before she could begin to pick up the shattered remains of life and carry on. I did not allow myself to dwell on their granddaughter.

The enormity of what I do struck me then. It is truly difficult to reconcile doing what needs to be done and doing it well, with such a bad, unpredictable outcome. This was not a man about to die from injuries so severe as to be subjected to surgery with nothing to lose. The was a well man who broke his ankle on holiday and now he was dead and gone forever. It is hard not to feel at fault.

As my experience grew I became much more detached: patients were patients, they needed treatments which I provided to the highest standard, yet sometimes they did not survive. That is the nature of the business we are in. That is the nature of life.

23. The Gastric Band

The population is gradually becoming more and more overweight and it follows that more and more patients requiring operations are obese. I don't mean operations for weight loss, or bariatric surgery to give it its full name. Only a minority of obese patients have these operations including gastric bands and gastric bypass. Many many more present for a variety of more routine operations such as knee replacements, gall bladder removal, hernia repair, and appendicectomy which may not be related to their obesity but which are now most definitely complicated by it.

Procedures for weight loss are considered the last resort for many who are desperate to reduce their weight. No matter what reason is motivating them, every person putting themselves forward for such intervention has one common belief: life will better when they are slimmer. The realists in the group will acknowledge that losing weight will not solve all of life's problems and will not miraculously transform them into happy, healthy, miniature versions of their current selves, but it will be a move in the correct direction towards these goals.

So what if bariatric surgery does not meet these expectations?

Until I met a patient I'll call Gemma, I too, thought that life would be far superior following this type of surgery and the associated weight loss. Gemma was larger than life in all senses of the phrase. She was vivacious, dressed in strong colours, she had voluminous hair, and was extensively made up with bright pink lipstick and thick mascara. She could talk for Britain. Occasionally I do like to chat to patients a little more than is strictly necessary, particularly if I find them interesting and have enough time. That day I was pleased I had plenty of time to listen.

It was a routine pre-operative visit for a minor gynaecological procedure and I went through my usual questions. Any medical conditions? Any previous anaesthetics or operations?

'I've had a gastric band fitted', she said.

An empty stomach is vitally important before anaesthesia to prevent passive regurgitation and aspiration of its contents. I was considering the relevance of her having a stomach the size of a walnut to my plan, when she continued.

''It's the worst thing I ever did you know' she paused for the first time during our consultation.

I looked up.

'What is, losing all that weight?'

'No,' she said, 'Getting the gastric band put in.'

She had weighed over 20 stones a year ago and was now a mere 13 stones, thanks to her 'band' as she called it.

I was surprised by her statement. Most people are much happier having lost such a significant amount of weight. I assumed everyone would be. Why ever not? My surprise must have shown.

'Oh, it was great at first' she said, 'There was a definite high as weight started to come off. The numbers went down, my clothes became too big and the compliments were rolling in. I even persuaded my mum and my sister to go and have a band fitted too. But then it changed'.

'In what way?' I asked, genuinely bewildered and interested to hear.

'Well, I started to become normal.'

Privately I thought this might be aspirational for the morbidly obese but this clearly was not a positive change for her.

'No-one stares at me in the swimming pool any more, I can now shop in high street stores rather than from out-sized catalogues, I can talk about diets like everyone else at work, yet I'm miserable' she continued.

'Really, in what way?' I was truly surprised.

'Every way!' she exclaimed and launched into the difficulties she now had.

'I LOVE food and I can't eat it! The band has left me with no choices. I can't choose to have a day off the diet or decide to allow myself one chocolate bar. I physically cannot accommodate the food anymore. Socialising, or even just going out is difficult now I can't eat from a buffet, I can't enjoy a canapé, and I can't grab a quick sandwich if I'm out shopping at lunch time. I'm restricted to smooth, sloppy, baby like food that will fit through the band. It's almost impossible to go out for dinner. If I see another bowl of carrot and coriander soup I will be tempted to drown myself in it! I used to be the centre of attention for all sorts of reasons but now I just blend in. I look the same as everyone else; a bit overweight and usually wearing black trousers, heels and the same party top as at least two other people in the room. I have become completely unremarkable.'

I was stunned by her revelations. I believed a gastric band to be an easy solution to a difficult problem. I believed feeling full on so little food and being unable to overeat would bring about weight loss that would solve more problems than it created. It seemed in life as well as in medicine, things are never quite straight forward.

It is easy to forget there are individuals behind the population guidelines. A normal body mass index (BMI) of 25 may not be the Holy Grail of dieting for the entire overweight population. Morbid obesity undoubtedly carries many great health risks, but then so does chronic, deep unhappiness. These problems may be less visible but are no less important.

There are very few obese people whom I believe to be truly happy with their size, despite their protestation to the contrary, but I think Gemma may be one of them.

24. Psychic Predictions

Four years into my training, I was reminded of the reading from the psychic lady I had as a medical student. Although I had not excelled (or even enjoyed) psychiatry as she predicted, I was reminded of something else she said; her vision of me being on a stage.

'So you're into drama and theatre?' she mused

'Oh no, not me.' I said quickly. She'd definitely got that wrong. 'My flatmate is though', I said optimistically, giving her an 'out'. My flatmate was the daughter of a major television star and was deep into theatre studies and film making. Close, I thought. Maybe she did have something. I gave her the benefit of the doubt and she kept trying.

'No, it's definitely you I'm seeing here. It's very clear, and it's not anyone else' she insisted, 'the stage is all set, I can see the curtains draped at the sides of the stage. They are not the usual burgundy velvet type, these look like seaweed. Dark, very strange looking. And you're late! Everyone is there, waiting for you. They need you to get there before they can start. It seems you're in charge of the show? I don't quite understand it. Does this mean anything to you?' she enquired hopefully, 'Think hard' she instructed, 'I can only convey what I'm seeing, what I'm feeling, what I'm sensing. I can't always explain it or know how to interpret it'.

'No,' I replied, 'Sorry. I've never been into anything like that in my life', I said shaking my head. I felt as if I was letting her down but the truth is, I was the least likely thespian I knew! I willed her to move on and tell me something, anything, about me and my future so I could justify her hefty fee from my limited student funds.

To say I was sceptical of fortune tellers was an understatement and I had been deliberately reticent throughout, giving away nothing that would allow inference. I had misled and misinformed and made the poor woman's job even harder, I imagined. After all, if she was so good at fortune telling the future she should hardly need to ask me any questions, yet she had. Was I a student? (I might be.) Had I managed to park easily? (Seemed an innocent question but I knew she was trying to trick an answer from me that would confirm I had a car, had driven to the appointment, could afford a car and would draw conclusions from that. I answered with a shrug.) She hadn't mentioned the fact that I had arrived late for my appointment. I had stopped for petrol on the way, the gauge was teetering above the red and I have a chronic anxiety about running out of petrol. The stop off had made me even later. But perhaps she already knew that?

At length she had made me reveal I was a medical student. We were at the end of the third year. It had been our first clinical year. Yes it was fascinating, a privilege. No we didn't mind the long hours (hadn't really thought about them at that stage), no I didn't know which branch of medicine I would go into.

'You will excel in psychiatry', she announced confidently. How she could tell when she'd only just discovered I was a medical student was beyond me. Maybe it was because only the mentally deranged would part with their hard earned cash to a woman with no qualifications purporting to see and tell the future?

Back in real life, the next term came and went. Psychiatry did nothing for me except make me feel sorry for those genuinely affected by bizarre delusions. It was not the specialty for me, of that I was sure.

Several years later I was reminded of my trip to the fortune teller. I was, by this time an anaesthetic registrar. One night on call I was fast bleeped to maternity theatre.

'Crash section, we need a quick GA, fetal heart's slowing', the obstetric registrar barked, as I entered the theatre. He was already scrubbed and holding the knife. The patient was lying on the operating table being given oxygen through a mask by the ODP in anticipation of my arrival. My drugs had all been prepared for me too, I noted them laid out neatly on the anaesthetic machine. The patient's abdomen was already cleaned and draped.

In an instant I registered the situation.

The surgical drapes were dark green and covered the patient liberally before flowing down to the floor. Similar material, the colour of seaweed covered the trolleys holding the instruments. The surgical team were gowned up in green gowns. The stage was set. Everyone was ready. Everyone had their own role. Everyone was looking at me, waiting for me, so they could begin.

As I induced anaesthesia it occurred to me that maybe there was something in this fortune telling business. This was my theatre and the stage was set for me, yet who could possibly have known that all those years before?

25. The Little Things

Sometimes as an anaesthetist you only see the worst parts of every department in the hospital. You never see a baby delivered normally. You rarely see healthy children. You do not see patients who are cured from their cancer. Instead you see complicated inductions of labour and fetal distress, delivery of newborns with holes in the heart or hernias which require early operation and you see many present in a pit of despair with their newly diagnosed cancer. In intensive care one in four of your patients will die despite your best efforts and on labour ward, severe pain will cause social graces to be thrown aside as patients curse and swear before feeling aghast and remorse. You will be asked to anaesthetise upset women for termination of pregnancy when your colleagues claim a moral reluctance to do so and you will provide an identical service for upset women who have suffered miscarriages (this time your colleagues would oblige too). Luckily the porters feel no such moral dilemma when wheeling these ladies down to theatre.

The theatre days are long with only a dim light at the end of the list. With no time to pop out for a cup of tea between patients we develop an innate ability to manage glucose level and fluid balance in the anaesthetic room, observing the patient's vital signs on the monitors in theatre through a glass panels in the door.

I often wish I could wear nice clothes at work. Go dressed in a smart suit as do lawyers and accountants, so I could feel like a true professional. Instead, most of my time is spent in baggy, unflattering theatre blues, indistinct from everyone else wearing baggy blues. (Blues make thin people look fat and fat people look fatter.)

I have to keep reminding myself that if I am bored during an operation then it's because things are going smoothly and without incident. This is a good thing.

This reality of hospital medicine makes times when a life is truly saved all the more memorable.

At the end of my first two years of training I had passed my exam and was about to move on to a registrar post. My last on call was with Dr Grange, a senior trainee who was about to be interviewed for a consultant post in the same department we were both currently working in. He had been on his best behaviour during the last year and of late was particularly keen to impress.On call his goal was to leave the boss in bed. It would show he could cope and would gain him some brownie points too.

Early in the evening a patient with a known, inoperable, laryngeal tumour in his throat presented acutely stridulous: his breathing noisy and sinister and he was clearly distressed. He could not speak such was his concentration on maximising each breath. The problem was that he time he breathed in, the tumour was drawn into the opening of his airway, blocking it to any further airflow. As he tried harder to breath, the worse it became. There were signs of in drawing, regression of the tissues around his neck and clavicles such was his effort of breathing. This had now progressed to a stage where breathing was ineffective and inadequate, and he required emergency access to his windpipe through the front of his neck to allow a route for breathing to occur bypassing the tumour above.

He was rushed from the ambulance straight to theatre.

He was dishevelled, with sparse but long greasy hair. He was wearing only brown trousers and a vest, both stained and far from fresh. His socks had holes at the toes. (Where were his shoes? Perhaps he left in too much of a hurry?)

Anyway, he was unconcerned by his appearance, having far more pressing problems that were consuming all his concentration.

Dr Grange and I were ready. He was pacing around going over the plan. I was excited; this was high stakes, a true matter of life and death balanced precariously on a knife edge. I was again glad I was not in charge of the procedure as Dr Grange thought aloud: the surgeons were scrubbed and ready to operate in theatre, we would add some anaesthetic vapour into a tight fitting oxygen mask and allow him to breathe himself gently off to sleep. Taking over his breathing would make a bad situation critical, as squeezing a bag full of gas into the airway would push the tumour further into the narrowed inlet. Once deep enough Dr Grange would look into the airway and hopefully be able to see beyond the obstruction enough to pass the breathing tube through the cords. This would provide a secure airway while the surgeons operated on the front of the patient's neck to form a permanent air inlet.

It all sounded good.

'Shall we get the consultant here just in case?' I suggested.

Dr Grange would be a consultant himself the following week but tonight he wasn't and my thinking was the on call consultant was responsible for us and may at least want to know what we were doing and have the opportunity to get involved.

'No, we'll be fine. Don't look so worried! It'll be fun!' I admired his confidence.

It was not fun.

With the oxygen flows at maximum the patient began to breath the gas mixture. We knew the gaseous induction process would be slow due to his low volume, obstructed breathing pattern and, as it turned out, it was too slow.

At the very onset of anaesthesia the patient's airway relaxed. All the muscles in his throat and neck had been taut, straining to hold the tumour up and out of the air passage. Even slight relaxation had been enough to obliterate this innate mechanism preserving life.

First do no harm.

The tumour settled at the entrance to the lungs, completely blocking it. The patient's abdomen was going in and out frantically as he continually tried to breathe against the obstruction, but to no avail. Dr Grange lifted the jaw, flexing the neck and extending the head as much as possible, he inserted a plastic airway into the patient's mouth to keep the tongue forwards, off the back of the throat and out of the way. Replacing the mask, he squeezed the bag, but the chest did not rise. With such little reserve, the oxygen saturation began to fall, the progressive flattening of the bleep tone signifying dangerously low levels had been reached all too quickly.

Dr Grange used both his hands to clamp the mask tightly to the patient's face and used his shoulder to wipe sweat from his face.

I leant against the oxygen flush button sending 40 litres per minute of oxygen into the bag. I screwed the pressure relief valve down tight so when I squeezed it, all the air was directed into the airway. A high pressure was needed if anything was to be achieved yet I suspected this was compounding the problem and wedging the tumour further in. Dr Grange still held on to the mask, as if clinging to it for his own life.

'Squeeze the bag!' he instructed. I squeezed but the chest did not rise. I squeezed again as the numbers continued to fall. It is possible that such pressurised, high volume oxygen flow can insufflate the lungs despite the lack of breathing and prolong the demise, but if this was happening it was not apparent.

The patient's colour changed from white to blue to an ominous grey. His heart rate, excessively high from the stress of breathing, now slowed. And slowed; the terminal sign of oxygen starvation.

The ODP looked at me. I looked at Dr Grange. He yelled 'Get the surgeon in here now!'.

When access to the airway has failed from above it has to be established rapidly from below. We are trained to do this but with a practiced surgeon present with surgical skills far superior to our ad hoc ability, it is quicker and more effective for them to do what they know best.

The surgical registrar did not rush. He came through the door, bewildered as he took in the scene, clearly shocked as he pieced together the situation, still wondering why he was needed in the anaesthetic room.

There was no time for pondering.

'Get on and do the trachy NOW' Dr Grange instructed him.

Still he did not move. His mouth opened to reply but no words came out. He began to stutter.

Dr Grange asked for the scalpel from the surgical tray and in a single movement slashed through the front of the moribund patient's neck. As a sea of blood poured out, he maneuvered our breathing tube through the hole he had made and into the airway.

With shaking hands slippery from the blood we fumbled to connect the oxygen system to the tube. Still the blood poured down both sides of the neck, covering the hands, all of them, desperately hanging onto the tube, to prevent it being dislodged in the panic.

Again I squeezed the bag, this time smearing it with blood. The patient's chest rose and fell and I enjoyed the feeling in my hand of the air recoiling and refilling the bag. It was indeed going in and out. Gradually the tone of the beeps increased, becoming tuneful again. As the oxygen in the circulation was restored so his colour returned. As his heart climbed back to normal, my own settled down. The scrub nurse shouted 'HE'S ALIVE! HE'S ALIVE!' for once not caring that the instruments were no longer sterile and the walls were spattered with blood 'HE'S ALIVE. YOU SAVED HIM! HOORAY!'. Such a show of positive emotion from the usually miserable nurse was unusual and illustrated the relief we all felt.

As the surgeon began to suture the bleeding veins in the neck I looked at Dr Grange. He didn't have to say a word despite being hailed the hero of the day by the nursing staff, despite the congratulations and remarks of respect and awe flying his way. I knew his career had flashed before his eyes. He knew he should have spoken to our consultant at the beginning. I met his eyes and knew then, that he knew, he had escaped by the skin of his teeth snatching the patient's life from the jaws of death at the very last second.

I had a little sympathy for him, although he was about to become a consultant and should be able to handle these emergencies. I was about to begin my next stage of training. In five years time that would be me, taking responsibility when it really mattered. I just hoped I felt up to it by then.

26. The Theatre of Theatre

The operating theatre, like any theatre, is a place for spectacle and showmanship. Historically, theatre was derived from Victorian freak shows, and later evolved into what we understand the word 'theatre' to mean today. As medical, surgical and anaesthetic practice advanced between 1840 and 1890, it was common for procedures to take place in an open lecture hall with an invited audience, there to ooohh and aaahh, and generally be impressed by the display of excellence. As the properties of ether as an anaesthetic agent 'able to render patients unconscious of torture' was discovered, a crowd again gathered to witness this display of magic, as it was considered. Only seeing was believing.

Patient safety is an important topic and has now risen to the top of the agenda . In recent years, we begin our day in theatre with a huddle. This involves the whole theatre team 'taking five' (not for a Twirl though) to run through the days list, making sure everyone knows the plan and is singing from the same hymn sheet. The purpose is to focus our thoughts and actions, to make sure everyone knows who each other is and that *everyone* feels empowered to speak up if they have *any* concerns. This will ultimately improve patient safety. No one can argue that it is a great idea and this is borne out in evidence from around the globe. What astounds me is how quickly it all goes out of the window as soon as the operation gets underway.

While I concede anaesthetising for a four hour ear operation is not the most riveting part of my week, there remains an element of theatre in theatre during such cases. These longer cases of highly complex surgery which require often very simple anaesthesia, can be a welcome relief from a busy list with fast and high levels of patient turnover for all members of the theatre team. I can pass the time quietly catching up on my journal reading and colouring in my chart with dots and seagulls, keeping my voice as low as the blood pressure and the patient suitably still and asleep. I keep an eye on the dismally slow progress of the operation via the television screen which is transmitting (live!) from the camera on the surgeon's headlight. This allows all interested parties in theatre to observe and admire the finer points of surgery from a safe distance. However, on looking around the theatre, it is clear there are few, if any, interested parties today.

Theatre sister, she who is charged with running the operating list smoothly, is lying on the floor, looking at the ceiling, both legs placed vertically against the wall. She withdraws from her trance-like state to inform us she is practicing Callanetics.

The senior staff nurse, scrubbed to assist the surgeon, looks redundant as he continues to focus down the microscope into the ear canal. She asked for a stool, sat down, then glanced around her instrument trolley looking for something else to keep her entertained. Bone wax is a material that looks like plasticine and can be moulded into shapes in much the same way. She had finished moulding it into a family of small Morph-like characters, all appropriately prodded with the instrument tips to make indentations for the eyes, nose and mouth. She was now using the surgeon's new dissection scissors to cut out shapes from a pile of swabs lying unused on the trolley. Animals, fish, trees; she had created some amazing topiary which would open out to unveil her efforts like a christmas decoration.

The surgical registrar, watching and learning, was showing the auxiliary staff how to line up their fingers in front of their face, go crossed eyed and visualise a floating sausage. (No, I'd never heard of this either) and the house officer had done the computing and the forms and was now sampling music from his smartphone. The same ones that might interfere with medical equipment.

The circulating nurse had won the coveted place at the computer and was googling cheap flights to Majorca for her 50th birthday celebration. Another was queueing to check out the shades of eye shadow now fashionable and expressed horror that no-one else changed their usual regime or 'look' each season.

The surgeon generally had to ask for his next instrument three times before anyone stopped in their tracks to realise that yes, he was talking to them. I wondered if this was what was really meant by the surgical pause.

But rest assured, as the end of the operation approached a professional air returned. Just as when the pilot announces 'cabin crew ten minutes to landing', suddenly everybody was awake and the noise level rose as we began to prepare, to tidy up, to get the dressings for the wound and a bed to transfer the patient onto at the end of the operation. I put my paperwork to one side and stood up, the best indicator of an anaesthetist paying attention. As the surgeon finished and left the table, it was 'cabin crew seats for landing' as we returned our focus to the patient and on waking him up safely.

The End.

I hope you enjoyed this book about my experience as a junior trainee in anaesthesia. If you did, you might consider leaving a review on the Amazon website. I would love to hear your thoughts and experiences too so please feel free to contact me at <u>drelliemay@gmail.com</u>

Look out for some more adventures in anaesthesia out soon.

CPSIA information can be obtained at www.ICGtesting.com
Printed in the USA
LVOW11s0244210815

450917LV00001B/31/P